# The Ultimate Guide to Anal Sex for Men

**BILL BRENT**

Illustrated by Zanne and Fish

CLEIS
PRESS

Published in the United States by Cleis Press Inc., P.O. Box 14684,
San Francisco, California 94114.

Printed in the United States.
Cover design: Scott Idleman
Book design: Karen Quigg
Cleis Press logo art: Juana Alicia
First Edition.
16 15 14 13

# Acknowledgments

Doug Harrison, for more than I can say.

Rob Stephenson, for the encouragement, inspiration, and friendly intimidation.

Lisa Montanarelli, whose eagle eyes have proofread—and improved—so much of my work. You are more than a friend and more than a colleague.

Jack Morin, Tristan Taormino, Bert Herrman, and all the others who have gone before me to lead the way to greater sexual pleasure and health. I list recommended books in Chapter Fourteen.

To my office staff, past and present—Lori, Selke, Jack Random, Doug Holland, and Tracey Darling—who put up with all the shenanigans I went through to complete this book: I love ya! A special thanks to Tracey for conducting most of the interviews.

Dr. Robert Lawrence, whose knowledge and sharing of time and resources have made this a better book. He is truly one of the unheralded heroes of the sexual revolution. Thanks to him and everyone else who lent me their reference books.

Tortuga Bi Liberty of Senior Unlimited Nudes (http://pages.prodigy.net/seniornude) for proofreading.

RedRight for his website, The RedRight Web (www.winternet.com/~redright/redright.html), and his input.

Helen Highwater (www.UnknownNews.net) for website-checking.

Kirk Read (www.kirkread.com) for the words of wisdom in Chapter 11.

Darklady (www.darklady.com) for help with Chapter 5.

Stuart and Tara Marcus, and Rob Jones, for giving me the time and the space.

Bob Mason and Clay Carman, for being my "L.A. Connection."

Lupe, for that incredible first time in the van.

Felice Newman, for giving me this chance.

Xaviera Hollander (aka The Happy Hooker), who first gave me the idea that sex could be crazy good fun.

My parents, who didn't mind my reading Xaviera Hollander's memoirs when I was a teen!

Everyone who took my written survey, and especially the ones who volunteered to talk with me and Tracey on the phone about their experiences. You represent the future of anal sex.

# Contents

## Illustrations

# Not in *My* Ass: 12 Myths about Anal Sex for Men

*I read somewhere that 30% of married couples had experimented with butt play or did it regularly. When you can recite statistics, people get this relieved look on their faces, like, "Oh, I'm not bad!" So I think there's a stigma, but it's what people think everybody else thinks, not necessarily what everybody else does think. I think that there's a ton more butt play going on than anybody's willing to admit.*

Most myths about anal sex are based on taboo. A taboo is an activity or object that is forbidden, usually without justification. Early in life we are trained to respect the anal taboo, which tells us that our anuses are disgusting, that we should tune out our awareness of our anus as much as we can, not become familiar with it, and certainly not think of our own anus as a source of pleasure.

## Myth #1: Anal Sex Is Unnatural and Immoral.

**Truth:** "Unnatural" and "immoral" are subjective terms that vary widely from culture to culture, as well as within a culture. What's considered "natural" and "moral" also shifts, according to the taste of the times. Oral sex, masturbation, and doggie-style penis/vagina intercourse were once considered deviant sexuality, as were sex outside of marriage and same-sex eroticism of any kind.

Trying to control or curb sexual expression is what's really unnatural. A healthier approach is to accept your sexual urges as part of an integrated, creative, self-aware existence. And most of us could admit to sexual desires that are politically incorrect. This is part of what makes sex fun and exciting for us. In fact, many people are attracted to anal sex precisely because it *is* so taboo and mysterious.

Thus, the only unnatural sex act is the one you can't do. Are men who can suck their own penises committing an unnatural act? How about women who can climax without touching themselves or being touched? Or enjoy seemingly unlimited orgasms? Whether it's due to luck or training, there is nothing "wrong" with such behavior.

## Myth #2: Nothing Was Meant to Go in There.

**Truth:** This myth is based on the idea that the only acceptable penetration is penis into vagina. Most of us can learn to relax the anus to accept a finger, penis, or sex toy, just as we can learn to relax the throat's gag reflex for fellatio or learn to be multiorgasmic.

The anus and rectum are capable of a tremendous degree of expansion and relaxation. *You can learn to consciously relax and expand the anus.* Desire is the most important element to success, and you can't fake this with anal sex. Here's a hint: Most people initially think that enjoyable anal sex is a matter of "controlling" the process, whereas it's really more about learning to let go and release. Surgeons often place their entire hands into anesthetized patients during rectal operations. While this is an extreme example—and I'm certainly not proposing anesthesia as a preparation for anal sex!—it does show that a relaxed body is capable of dilating the anal sphincter to a tremendous degree.

Anal pleasure is achievable for almost everyone who's motivated by their own enjoyment. Jack Morin, author of *Anal Pleasure and Health,* has worked with hundreds of people who wanted to enjoy anal sex. He observes that motivation strongly influences success, and he distinguishes between performance and pleasure-oriented goals. Of his patients who completed therapy, those who did it to please their partners had a success rate of roughly 66%. However, where patients were working with Morin for their own enjoyment, the success rate went up to 89%.[1]

## Myth #3: The Anus Was Never Intended to Be Eroticized.

**Truth:** Says who? That's like saying that squash was never meant to be eaten since it has to be cooked first. And who's more likely to be correct: the folks who are familiar with squash and know how to prepare it, or the folks who remain ignorant about it yet denounce everyone who likes it?

Like the head of the penis, the anal region is rich in nerve endings. In fact, some men experience intensely pleasurable sensations in the penis during receptive anal penetration. The prostate gland, an important sexual organ that can only be stimulated directly through anal penetration, is a source of great pleasure for many men.

Women also experience intensely pleasurable sensations during anal sex. Like the clitoris, the nerve-rich anus can transmit subtle sensations. Some women report that anal sex provides G-spot stimulation. The vagina and the rectum share a common wall, and that area can enjoy being stimulated as well. In fact, the nerves are closer to the anal side of the wall, making the sensations different and sometimes stronger. Some women even enjoy stimulating both sides of the wall simultaneously.

The perineal region (the area between the vagina and anus in women and between the scrotum and anus in men) can provide its own delight when stimulated during anal sex.

Like the genitals, the anus engorges with blood during sex and contracts upon orgasm. Some people learn to control these contractions to prolong orgasm and increase its intensity.

See Chapter Two, "How It Works, and How to Work It," for more information on both male and female anorectal anatomy.

## Myth #4: The Bible Says It's Wrong.

**Truth:** Many assertions of this nature stem from a misinterpretation of the book of Leviticus, in which the towns of Sodom and Gomorrah are burned to the ground allegedly because of "unnatural" sexual acts (hence the term "sodomy"). Actually, though, the towns were burned to punish their residents *not* for indulging in sodomy but rather for behaving inhospitably to strangers.

## Myth #5: Anal Sex Is Dirty and Messy.

**Truth:** This taboo is based on the fact that the intestine is an organ of elimination, and that what comes out is smelly. However, reasonable hygiene corrects this situation. Also, condom and glove use go a long way toward making anal sex hygienic and more pleasurable as well.

A healthy digestive system normally empties the rectum when it eliminates waste. Usually only trace amounts of feces remain in the rectum. A diet with sufficient fiber can help avoid messy bowel movements. We'll cover this in Chapter Four, "Hygiene and Diet."

Most people who like anal sex wash the anal region and genitals before play. A soapy shower or bath before anal sex, perhaps using antibacterial soap, removes any residual bacteria that can cause smells. Some people like those smells, though, and there's nothing wrong with that. There are also various ways of cleaning your anal passage internally, if you want to go that far.

## Myth #6: Anal Sex Is Painful for the Recipient, Who Only Receives to Please His (or Her) Partner.

**Truth:** With the addition of lubricant, a relaxed anus can be entered without pain or discomfort.

It's a common belief, even among people who are very experienced with anal sex, that anal sex must hurt initially before it gets comfortable enough to enjoy. This is not true. When you feel discomfort, your anal sphincters are telling you to back off. If you plunge ahead anyhow, you can hurt yourself, which can make your body more tense and even more resistant to future experimentation.

Sometimes, when the sphincters resist painful anal stimulation (that is, when they go into anal spasm), the muscles eventually surrender. Often this is accompanied by the cessation of pain, which some people mistake for pleasure when it's actually just the sphincters giving up and numbing out. Pleasuring an anus with a sphincter that starts out relaxed and stays relaxed throughout is, in fact, a very different and vastly more pleasurable experience.

Many of us, especially men, subscribe in varying degrees to the motto of "No Pain, No Gain." We get all tangled up in cultural ideas about masculinity and pain, to the point where the two may become indistinguishable. The culmination of this mentality is clearly spelled out in another motto, the exhortation to "take it like a man" (which has some ironic implications regarding masculinity where receptive anal and oral sex are concerned!). The assumption here is that enduring pain is part of what it takes to be a real man (which must mean that women who bear children are the butchest men of all!), and that tolerating pain somehow makes us more masculine.

So while "No Pain, No Gain" might be a useful mantra for weightlifting, it won't serve you when it comes to enjoying anal sex. This pain-enduring mindset can get in the way of pleasurable anal sex because it implies that anal sex is something that must be endured rather than enjoyed. Well, guys, anal sex does *not* have to hurt. If you or your partner experience any pain, it's a cue to stop, evaluate what's going on, and make any necessary adjustments, up to and including stopping altogether.

Some people enjoy the endorphin rush of pain endurance as part of their sexual play, and if that's your scene, fine—but we're addressing something else here. The point is that no one should ever have to endure anal pain to please a partner. Many people have learned to relax and enjoy butt play, alone and with a partner, and you can become one of them. It's your sexual right not to engage in any behavior that causes you discomfort, and it's your obligation to yourself to speak up when this occurs. Anal sex doesn't ever have to hurt.

## Myth #7: Anal Sex Is Harmful and Physically Dangerous.

**Truth:** Some people fear that if they engage in receptive anal sex, their anus will eventually lose its elasticity, leading to incontinence and the need to wear diapers. Actually, stretching the sphincter and rectal tissue safely over time tends to strengthen rather than loosen the muscles associated with anal sex, as people who practice fisting and using large toys can attest. It's just like exercising the muscles in any other part of your body.

The most physically dangerous thing you can do to your anorectal region is to put something up your butt that shouldn't be there. There are two ways this may happen: (1) Trying to insert too much too quickly, such as a hand or a toy. Fortunately, we have an excellent auto-feedback system in the form of pain. Quite simply, if you are doing something that hurts, then stop doing it. (2) Inserting foreign objects, especially anything that's breakable, or anything with a sharp edge or a point, whether exposed or hidden. Scratching the rectal walls can lead to perforation, which can result in peritonitis, which is fatal if not treated promptly.

It's also dangerous to insert anything that doesn't have a flange (flared base) or a cord—that is, anything that has nothing you can use to pull it out—because objects without handles can get sucked up into the anal cavity, making removal potentially difficult. Usually, such objects will eject themselves if you squat patiently and relax while taking deep breaths.

Another major risk factor is abusing drugs in conjunction with anal sex. I'll have more to say on this later, particularly in Chapters Twelve and Thirteen, but the bottom line (no pun intended) is this: If you have to get high to do it, then don't do it. In particular, if you feel you need to take a drug to dampen the pain involved with a sexual act, then you're not doing it right. Drug use can impair judgment and lead to accidents.

## Myth #8: Anal Sex Is the Easiest Way to Get AIDS.

**Truth:** Viruses can be transmitted through anorectal tissue, which is highly absorbent and can be easily torn. Unprotected anal intercourse with an HIV-positive person *is* a high-risk activity regardless of who is the insertive partner, although recent studies show that it's statistically much easier to transmit the virus to the receptive partner than to the insertive one.

But when engaged in with knowledge, protection, and communication, anal sex is considered a low-risk sexual activity. Partners who are both HIV-negative (as tested six months after the last contact with a potentially HIV-positive person or their infected bodily fluids) can have unprotected anal intercourse without risk of infection. Partners who are both HIV-positive may be at risk of reinfection with a variant strain of the virus if they carry differing strains of the virus and engage in anal intercourse without protection. Safer sex practices can help prevent transmission of HIV and other STDs. I will explore safer sex techniques in Chapter Six, "Latex and Lube."

## Myth #9: Only Gay Men Do It.

**Truth:** Our culture erroneously assumes that virtually all gay men regularly engage in anal sex. Since we have an intercourse-centered view of sex, this assumption is natural, if unfortunate. Since the only "real" sex in our culture is intercourse—and since the only intercourse available between two men is anal—then, by this myth, anal intercourse must be the gay version of vaginal intercourse among heterosexuals.

While reports and studies over the past decade on the prevalence of anal sex among gay men vary widely, it's clear that many gay men never engage in anal sex and many straight couples love anal sex. In fact, nowadays the fastest-growing group of anal aficionados may be heterosexual couples. According to Susie Bright, "It's ironic: even though butt-fucking is popularly associated with gay men in today's sexual culture, it is in fact heterosexuals who have gone wild about their asses. Ask anyone who works in a sex toy shop what single item has surged forward in sales in the past fifteen years: butt plugs. And dildo harnesses for women who are clearly involved with men."[2]

Contrary to stereotype, anal sex is also popular among lesbians. A recent study of lesbian and bisexual women found that 50% reported having anal sex with women during the prior year.[3]

Nonetheless, the current generation of anal sex aficionados owes a debt to the gay male sex culture that evolved during the 1970s, which popularized and, to some extent, demystified the practice of anal sex. Thanks to their explorations, nowadays more of us know more about anal sex and what it involves than our parents and grandparents did.

## Myth #10: Straight Guys Who Do Anal Are Really Gay.

**Truth:** This is an extension of the previous myth. That this continues to be a strong belief attests to the anal taboo's enduring power. By their very nature, taboos transcend reason and logic.

If you're heterosexual and you like it when your girl-friend sticks a lubricated pinkie up your butt, well, that doesn't mean that you will forsake her and only put men's fingers up your butt henceforth. If she straps on a big, greasy dildo and rides you until your vision blurs, that doesn't mean that you're going to embark on a quest for the perfectly hung man. Wanting a woman to play with your butt doesn't make you any less straight than some unimaginative clod who humps his wife's pussy for fifteen seconds and shoots his load. And who's having more fun?

Jack Morin says: "I get letters from all over the world thanking me for writing about anal sex, and one of the biggest subgroups is from straight guys who say, 'I'm so glad I'm not the only one who loves this stimulation—I've always wanted to tell my partner about it...but I've worried in the back of my mind that this means I'm gay, even though I'm not attracted to men.'"[4]

Everyone, whether gay, straight, bisexual, transgendered, or whatever, has a butt—and every butt can provide pleasurable sensations when given the opportunity.

## Myth #11: Recipient Males Are Weak or Secretly Want to Be Women.

**Truth:** This taboo is based in part on the belief that sexual receptivity is exclusively feminine.

Men can view anal receptivity as humiliation or surrender, and this can block enjoyment. Receptivity is actually an extremely active and powerful experience: Both emotionally and physiologically, it can be very demanding and profound. It's a statement that you accept someone else's presence within your body. Some people find that it's the most intense sexual experience they can have. Quite often, men who enjoy anal receptivity have had to overcome a lot of negative social conditioning that tells them they're bad for wanting and enjoying this. Does that sound "weak" to you?

Virile men of all orientations enjoy receptive anal sex. Still, many men are afraid of being perceived as womanly because they enjoy being the recipient. Even some gay men who love being penetrated, or even just fantasizing about it, believe that doing so makes them less of a man. Such internalized homophobia and misogyny is worth overcoming.

It's healthy to explore your own attitudes about this. If you asked a roomful of people, perhaps teenagers, "What's wrong with being a gay man? What's wrong with being womanly or feminine?," you would realize how deeply and unconsciously many of us have internalized some of society's negative attitudes toward women and gay men. You would further realize that these attitudes are based on fear rather than reason. If a man allows this fear to stop him from enjoying an activity that's rightfully his to enjoy, then it is he, not the man who's enjoying himself, who is the weak one.

Recognize that each of us is a unique mixture of masculine and feminine components, that neither is inherently better than the other, and that appreciating this range within ourselves promotes acceptance of others and their uniqueness.

## Myth #12: Only Perverts and Sluts Do It.

**Truth:** Well, this myth is true and not true. Many people eroticize themselves or their partners as "perverts" or "sluts" during sex. There's nothing pathological about this behavior, and in fact such role-playing can be healthy and fun. Actually, there's nothing more inherently perverse about anal sex than there is about oral sex (or any other form of sex), but hey, if it makes you hot *thinking* that there is, please don't let me deflate your hard-on.

"Pervert" is usually invoked as a slur against someone who engages in sex that others fear or don't understand. When we're ignorant about a variant form of sex, many of us will deride it to avoid revealing our own fear and ignorance, or perhaps to mask our own curiosity. It's important to be a bit dispassionate about passion— remember that the word "sex" has three conjugations: "*I* am differently pleasured; *you* are kinky; *he* is a pervert."

A "slut" is a promiscuous person—in common parlance, almost always a woman or a gay man. So why are promiscuous straight men lauded as studs while everyone else is denigrated as a slut? This is a clue that, as with Myth #1, some people are eager to play the voice of authority and hold their value judgments over others.

In some sexual subcultures, "pervert" and "slut" have been reclaimed as badges of sexual and personal power, as has happened already with other slurs such as "queer" and "bitch." In fact, an excellent book, called *The Ethical Slut*,[5] makes a strong case for nonmonogamy as a healthy lifestyle choice when combined with effective communication and a loving attitude toward one's primary partner.

In any case, there's no logical, cause-and-effect relationship between promiscuity and anal sex. In fact, while some people *do* engage in anal sex with a variety of partners, many others reserve anal sex for one special person. Neither is inherently better or worse, nor more or less moral. And finally, the reverse is true: Learning to enjoy anal sex won't turn you into a slut, either, although it may make you want to have more anal sex!

**EXERCISE** ▶ **Make a List**

What are your fears regarding anal intimacy? Make a list. Don't worry if you sound silly or uptight. If you have a partner, you can ask him or her to do the same. Tuck the list away until you finish with this book, then review it to see if your fears have lessened or changed.

Naming fears can be an effective way to deal with them. Giving a scary behavior a name reduces its power over us; by facing our fears, we can begin to break through them and open new opportunities for growth.

## NOTES

1. Jack Morin, *Anal Pleasure and Health: A Guide for Men and Women* (Down There Press, 1998).

2. Susie Bright as quoted in Tristan Taormino, *The Ultimate Guide to Anal Sex for Women* (Cleis Press, 1997), 17.

3. Jeanne M. Marrazzo as quoted in Felice Newman, *The Whole Lesbian Sex Book: A Passionate Guide for All of Us* (Cleis Press, 1999), 249. Marrazzo found that of the 149 women in her study, more than half had anal sex with women in the prior year. Slightly more than one-third had engaged in rimming in the prior year.

4. Jack Morin, as quoted on Sexuality.Org. Excerpt from a presentation, "Clinical Aspects of Anal Sexuality," which Morin delivered at a joint conference of the Society for the Scientific Study of Sexuality and the American Association of Sex Educators, Counselors, and Therapists (Nov. 11–15, 1998). www.sexuality.org/morin98.html

5. *The Ethical Slut: A Guide to Infinite Sexual Possibilities*, by Dossie Easton and Catherine Liszt (Greenery Press, 1998).

# How It Works, and How to Work It: Anatomy and Exercise

A basic understanding of anorectal anatomy will enhance your enjoyment of anal sex. Knowing how this system works will enable you to locate the muscles used in anal sex and will help you control and develop them to maximize your sexual pleasure. It will also give you some ideas for explaining what's going on "down there" to shy or nervous partners, which will reassure them and help them relax, with the goal of better sex for you both.

## Anorectal Anatomy

Anatomy as a field of science and medicine is at times surprisingly subjective, given to a variety of interpretations and opinions about the structure of the human body. This is particularly true regarding our sexual anatomy. Our discussion here is based on my interpretation of medical textbooks, sex manuals, numerous Internet resources, and conversations with sex educators.

For our purposes, we'll explore the three outermost areas of the large intestine: the anus, the rectum, and the descending colon (herein referred to as simply "the colon").

### The Anus

This is the anal canal's external opening of soft, pinkish tissue folds, which give it a puckered appearance. The anus is located several inches below the tailbone and several inches above the scrotum, directly behind the

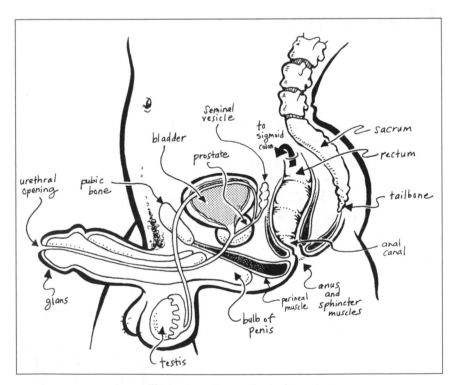

**Illustration # 1: Male Anatomy**

perineum. The anus is rich in blood vessels and sensitive nerve endings that enjoy stimulation and touch. The area surrounding the opening is populated with follicles; while every adult has hair surrounding the anus, it varies in appearance from fine and downy to thick and dark.

## The Anal Sphincters

The anal opening contains two sphincters. Although they're called "internal" and "external," they are actually somewhat overlapping bands of circular muscle.

The external sphincter is controlled by the central nervous system, which in turn controls all our voluntary muscles, such as those in our hands or legs. Typically, the external sphincter is under our control; it's the

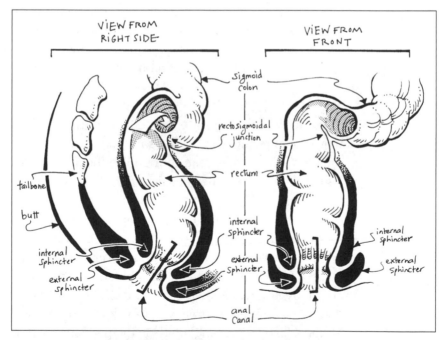

**Illustration # 2: Anorectal Anatomy**

muscle you tighten when it's time to poop but you can't expel immediately.

The internal sphincter, by contrast, is part of the autonomic nervous system, which controls reflexive functions such as breathing and blood pressure. With practice, one may learn to exert some degree of influence over the action of the internal sphincter. This seems to be the spot that stores up much of the tension and stress in the anal region, which can lead to hemorrhoids. Learning to relax the sphincters is valuable in terms of preventing or lessening the frequency of hemorrhoids and other anal discomfort.

A relaxed sphincter is capable of allowing feces to be expelled, whereas a tense sphincter is capable of excretion only by straining, if at all. Likewise, it's the tense state of the sphincters that makes anal penetration painful and difficult, whereas relaxed sphincters facilitate pleasurable, pain-free anal penetration. Shortly we'll explore some techniques for promoting anal relaxation.

**The Perineal Muscles**

Close to the sphincters are the perineal muscles, which have some relationship to the sphincters. The perineal muscles support the tissue surrounding the anus as well as the area between the genitals and the anus, called the perineum.

Two specific perineal muscles are important to our purposes. The first is the *bulbocavernosus* muscle. In men, it envelops the bulb (not to be confused with the head) of the penis, between the scrotum and the anus. This muscle serves to help empty the urethral canal after urination. After ejaculation, you can expel most residual seminal fluid by pressing firmly on the perineum, sliding your finger upward past the scrotum and along the underside of the shaft toward the urethral opening (meatus). You can feel the bulbocavernosus muscle by pressing on the approximate center of your perineum. You may feel a slight twinge, and your penis may jump a little. Most men find some pressure on this point to be pleasurable, while others experience discomfort.

The second important muscle is the *pubococcygeus muscle,* more commonly known as the "PC muscle." This muscle is the same one you use to stop the flow of urine while peeing. You can squeeze it while you're urinating or by simply pretending to urinate. You can feel the muscle contract by placing your finger on your perineum (the area between your genitals and your anus). Also, you can feel the contractions strongly in your anus. The PC muscle contracts randomly during sexual arousal and rhythmically during orgasm. Learning to control it voluntarily can enhance the quality of sex.

> "Orgasm happens in the brain. The closely associated set of pelvic physical responses are very often considered orgasm but are really a set of low lumbar and sacral reflexes."
> —DR. ROBERT LAWRENCE, SEX EDUCATOR[1]

To some degree, all orgasms are anal orgasms. The anal sphincters are connected to the pelvic floor running throughout the pelvis. The anus contracts at the same time and at the same rate as the other muscles involved in orgasmic contractions.

The PC muscle is part of a flat, supportive muscle system known as the *pelvic sling.* The pelvic sling anchors to the pubic bone on one side, wraps behind the back of the rectum, and anchors to the other side of the pubic bone. It has two functions: to support the rectum, and to assist us in holding back a bowel movement. While the external sphincter has some influence over this, it's mainly the job of the pelvic sling. It can become chronically tense;

when it contracts, it compresses the rectum. This is possibly a major cause of constipation as well as not being able to enjoy anal penetration. In "Techniques and Exercises," below, I will cover some techniques to help relax this muscle, which will enhance your anal pleasure.

## The Rectum and the Anal Canal

The rectum is about eight inches long and opens directly into the anal canal, which is about an inch long. Because of their flexibility and strength, the anus and the rectum can adapt to a wide range of variously sized and shaped penises, butt plugs, and dildos.

A rich and complex network of nerve endings extends all around the anal opening, as well as underneath the head of the penis. Stimulation of these nerve endings is chiefly responsible for the pleasure (or pain) experienced during anal sex. However, the rectum, like the vaginal walls, responds more to pressure than other sensations. Thus, the anal walls are not as surface-sensitive as the anal opening.

Contrary to popular belief, the rectum isn't a straight tube; in most people, it's S-shaped, meaning that there are two major curves along its length. Running into the rectal wall with a sex toy or a penis accounts for much of the internal discomfort felt in anal sex; I'll address that in Chapter Nine, which is dedicated to penetration.

## The Prostate Gland

An important male sexual organ, the prostate gland produces prostatic fluid, the lubricant that facilitates the ejaculation of sperm. Prostatic fluid is a whitish secretion and gives ejaculate its whitish appearance. It collects within the prostate and feeds into the urethra during ejaculation. Prostatic fluid makes up about one-third of the total ejaculate, along with sperm and seminal fluid. It helps sperm to swim and protects them from being damaged by the acidity of urine in the urethra.

The prostate lies just below the bladder and just in front of the rectum. You can find the prostate by placing your index finger all the way into the anus and pressing toward the front of the body along the rectal wall. It should be about two inches inside the anus. Rub gently and slowly, as any sudden hitting of the prostate can be painful. In a few men, it will cause spontaneous ejaculation.

A healthy prostate will feel like a lump the size of a small walnut, and the texture is similar to the ball of muscle at the V of the thumb and index finger when making a fist. The prostate enlarges during arousal, so it's easier to feel it then. The prostate gland is very sensitive to stimulation and can only be directly stimulated internally—that is, by inserting a finger, penis, or implement into the butt. When you're highly aroused, in the sustained plateau phase, you can rub it to see if you like the feeling or whether it affects your ejaculation.

## The Colon

Lying above the rectum is the colon. The two are separated by a curving junction called the *sigmoid*. Understanding the curve of this junction becomes important in more advanced forms of anal play such as fisting and penetration with large toys. When feces exit the colon into the rectum, the pressure triggers the rectal reflex. At this point, the *internal sphincter* automatically relaxes.

## The Large Intestine

Essentially, the large intestine is one continuous tube, approximately six feet long, comprising five sections—ascending colon, transverse colon, descending colon, sigmoid, and rectum—and ending at the anus. Its purpose is to absorb vitamins, minerals, and water, as well as to move digestive waste from the small intestine to the anus, where it's expelled. It's characterized by folds and curves. The folds give the large intestine a great degree of expansion, much like an accordion.

The large intestine is particularly efficient at liquid absorption, which turns the liquid waste of the small intestine into solid feces. (This absorptive quality, coupled with the delicacy of the anal tissue, is what makes the anorectal region particularly susceptible to infections transmitted via body fluids, such as HIV and gonorrhea.) The smooth muscles of the intestinal walls, combined with a lubricating lining of mucosal tissue, ensure the easy movement of bulky, solid waste through the large intestine.

## Techniques and Exercises

Many of us spend a lot of time keeping in shape, but few of us do anything specifically to strengthen the anogenital region. Doing a few simple exercises on a daily basis is easy. These exercises can be performed while doing other activities, plus you can get a big payoff in sexual enjoyment, as well as a tangible health benefit in the form of a strengthened pelvic region overall. This may aid in the prevention of sexual dysfunction and certain diseases such as prostate cancer.

### Kegel Exercises

The late gynecologist Arnold Kegel worked with his patients in the 1950s to develop a series of exercises to strengthen the PC and vaginal muscles. These exercises have become known simply as "Kegels." There are three exercises you can do, and you can do them almost anywhere, even while bathing, shopping, driving, or watching TV.

Kegels are easy to do, they feel good, they don't take any real time out of your day, and, best of all, they offer tangible sexual benefits. First, steady practice will enable both men and women to prolong and intensify orgasm and erotic sensations in general. Second, they can improve general sexual function in men as well as women. Strengthening the ability to clamp the PC muscles voluntarily is helpful in preventing premature ejaculation and is key to attaining male multiple orgasm. Kegels can also increase the strength of erections and probably even extend erectile function later in life. Women who do their Kegels sometimes discover an increase in their natural vaginal lubrication. Third, they're an excellent way to tone the pelvic region. Other muscles, including the sphincters, contract along with the PC muscle, which builds strength in the anal region and enables us to more fully enjoy anal play, particularly penetration. Lax, mushy muscles are not very sensitive, and they require excess tension to do their work. Firm, well-toned, yet relaxed soft muscle tissue in the pelvic region increases sexual sensitivity and responsiveness.

Finally, the exercises are a great stress reliever. You may find that regular practice gives you a more balanced, confident stance in the world. The deep breathing alone will help your entire body feel more open and alive.

EXERCISE #1:
Inhale deeply as you contract the PC muscles and clench them for a few seconds. Then exhale all the way and relax. Do 100 repetitions a day for best results; if the thought of so many reps overwhelms you, begin with fewer and work your way up. You can break them up into 3 or 4 sets and do them throughout the day.

EXERCISE #2:
Inhale deeply and as you do, clench and release the PC muscles quickly, 8 to 12 times per breath. Then exhale and relax. Do 20 to 50 sets a day.

EXERCISE #3:
Inhale and pretend you're sucking water into your anus and genitals. Then exhale and bear down, pushing out the imaginary water. This is great for your abdominal muscles as well. Do about 10 repetitions at a time, 1 to 3 times a day.

One variation on this exercise is to inhale with a pushing rather than a sucking motion of the anus and other pelvic muscles, followed by the sucking motion before exhaling with a complete release. An interesting note: Some people do develop the ability to suck up water into their rectum using this technique.

## Prostate Massage May Improve Health

Prostate cancer is the most common nonskin cancer found in American men and a leading cause of death among older men.[2] (Interestingly, the next most commonly diagnosed cancer in American men is colorectal cancer.) Increasing evidence shows that men who don't directly stimulate the prostate (particularly men who practice long-term sexual abstinence) are more vulnerable to prostate cancer and other prostate problems such as prostatitis (inflammation)[3] and benign prostatic hyperplasia (a noncancerous enlargement of the prostate).

Thus, every man should know how to find his prostate and how to massage it. This is a good example of that preventive medicine that HMOs are always touting, although you certainly won't find many of them discussing prostate massage! Yet prostate massage has been part of Asian medicine for centuries. In traditional Japanese families, wives often massage their husbands' prostate to promote prostatic health, a practice that the spouses and partners of Western men with prostate cancer are learning in mounting numbers.[4] Actually, it's easier for a partner to massage the prostate from behind because the angle is better and more of the finger is available.

At this point, the Western medical establishment knows little about the mechanics of prostate cancer, and much research remains to be done in this area. Thus, it behooves the patient to become better informed than most doctors. Apparently it's possible for some men to heal their prostate cancer; many books on the subject are available, and support groups and other resources can readily be found on the Internet. While many doctors frown on the use of prostate massage alone as cancer treatment, considering it risky in the absence of other medical intervention, anecdotal cases tell of remission following such therapy.[5] Advocates claim that consistent prostate massage improves the muscle tone of the prostate and helps drain the fluids that accumulate in cancer cases. While prostate cancer is very slow to progress (many patients die of other causes), treatment may improve one's quality of life.

### Massaging the Prostate Gland

Of course, we don't have to have prostate problems to enjoy the benefits of prostate massage. You can stimulate the prostate directly by placing a finger or implement into the butt. For this you'll need your index finger and some form of lubricant, plus a latex glove if you wish. One technique is to lie on your left side and put your right hand behind your back; reverse this if you're left-handed. It may be easier if you start with the top-most leg bent at the knee, toward the chest, and then straighten it after you are inside. Enter your rectum slowly, locate the prostate gland, and gently thrust and massage it. Be sure that you're not pushing too hard or poking at an angle. Exert firm pressure on the upper portion of the prostate, and slowly push downward and toward the middle. As the prostate is heart-shaped, it has two lobes. If you can feel them separately, you can massage one lobe and then the other. Otherwise, just apply any pressure that's not uncomfortable. Some strain on the wrist is normal, however. This tends to be easier to do if you're slim and flexible.

Here are a couple of alternative or supplementary techniques: Thrust in and out toward the anal sphincter, varying the rate to get maximum stimulation. Or use a vibrator on the sphincter to also stimulate a large number of nerve endings and indirectly stimulate the prostate. Another way to stimulate the prostate indirectly is to press and massage the perineum with your fingers. In Asian medicine, the perineum is an important acupressure point for good prostate health and sexual functioning.

Some men have trouble reaching their prostate or finding a partner to do it for them. For them, and for others interested, a device is available to massage the prostate and the perineum simultaneously, named the Pro-State Prostate & Perineal Prostate Massager. (The manufacturer's website states that "it is helpful to master the Kegel Method and to synchronize breathing,"[6] so doing those exercises clearly pays off here.)

Many men find that applying pressure to the prostate gland increases sexual pleasure and enhances orgasm. Others, however, find any pressure unpleasant no matter what they do. And yet other men enjoy prostate stimulation only after they have reached a certain level of sexual arousal. Individual reports of sensation vary widely, from ecstasy to mild pleasure to indifference to discomfort. So it's very much an individual preference.

## Female Anatomy

Why should a book about anal sex for men touch on female anatomy? Well, if you're having anal sex with a woman, there are a few things you need to know. With the exception of the prostate, female anorectal anatomy is the same as male anorectal anatomy—women possess the same nerve-filled, delicate tissue of the anus, the same curves and turns of the rectum, and so forth. But there *are* a few special things you'll need to know.

## G-Spot

The G-spot is a cushion of tissue wrapped around the urethra. A woman's urethral sponge can be stimulated through the front wall of the vagina, just as a man's prostate gland can be stimulated through the front wall of the rectum. In fact, numerous G-spot vibrators and vibrator attachments are available that are curved to hit just the right spot on the vaginal front wall.

As with prostate stimulation, a woman's reaction to G-spot stimulation can vary widely. Some women love G-spot stimulation, some find it irritating unless they're quite aroused, and others don't like it at all. Rear-entry vaginal penetration is the easiest method of finding and stimulating the G-spot. Anal penetration also stimulates the G-spot in some women, since the anal canal is so close to the vagina; in fact, they share a common wall. Many women ejaculate with G-spot stimulation, producing a clear fluid that either spurts or gushes from the urethra just before or during orgasm.

## Double Penetration

Some women enjoy the feeling of being filled simultaneously in both the vagina and the anus. While the anus can expand to accept a finger, penis, or dildo—or even a whole hand—the vagina stretches even more readily with arousal. Thus you may be able to penetrate your partner's vagina with your penis while her anus is still stretching to accommodate a pinky finger. Some women enjoy anal penetration with a finger or butt plug during vaginal pen-

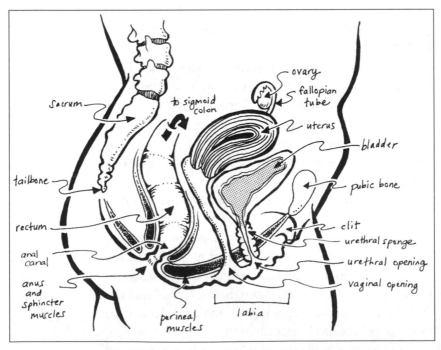

**Illustration # 3: Female Anatomy**

etration. The combinations are practically limitless. Porn is filled with images of double penetration, with one woman being penetrated by two penises. A flexible, double-headed dildo can be inserted into both of her orifices at once. The safest double dildos have a bulb in the middle designed to keep anal secretions away from the vagina. Which brings us to a few important precautions.

While oil-based lubricants may be preferred by some for anal play, they should *never* be used in the vagina. The vagina, unlike the anal canal, doesn't flush itself out daily, and the residual oil provides fertile ground for bacteria, leading to vaginal infections. It also is important to keep anal secretions—including lube and semen—away from the vulva. Anal secretions can transfer bacteria from the intestinal tract to the vagina, causing bacterial infections in both the vagina and the urinary tract.

So it's important to keep anything that has been in the anus away from the vagina until it has been thoroughly cleaned. See Chapter Seven, "Tools and Toys," for details on how to clean toys.

 **Rock Steady**

Start by slowly moving your hips forward and back, from side to side, and in a wide, comfortable circle. Try this before and after the pelvic exercises above. You'll probably feel more relaxed the second time you do this movement series. Practice relaxing and moving your pelvis more freely than usual any time you are moving throughout your day, whether walking, running, dancing, or doing other forms of exercise.

NOTES

1. Email correspondence between author and Dr. Lawrence, November 2001.

2. E. Silverberg, C. C. Boring, and T. S. Squires, Cancer Statistics, 1990. CA 1990; 40:9–26: R. Scott, D. L. Mutchnik, T. Z. Laskowski, and W. R. Schmalhorst. 1969. Carcinoma of the prostate in elderly men: Incidence, growth characteristics and clinical significance. *J Urol* 101:602–607: J. E. Montie, D. P. Wood, J. E. Pontes, J. M. Boyett, and H. S. Levin. 1989. Adenocarcinoma of the prostate in cystoprostatectomy specimens removed for bladder cancer. *Cancer* 63:381–85.

   See also www.a-urology.com/uro001.htm, an excellent, informative site. Fortunately, prostate cancer is the slowest-growing common cancer, and most men who contract prostate cancer die of other, presumably unrelated, causes.

3. *The Merck Manual of Medical Information*, Home Edition (see www.merck.com/pubs/mmanual_home/sec21/229.htm), recommends that "When prostatitis isn't caused by an infection, warm sitz baths (baths in which the person sits), periodic prostate massage, and frequent ejaculation are recommended to relieve symptoms."

4. An excellent page on prostate self-massage can be found at www.prostatitis.org/doityourself.html.

5. See, for example, www.prostate90.com/index.html

6. www.highisland.com. See Chapter Fourteen, "Resources," for complete contact and ordering information.

# Self-Exploration and Self-Play: Massage, Masturbation, and More

**Looking and Touching**

Many of us have never really looked at our own anuses. Doing so is an excellent and very safe way to start exploring anal play. Becoming familiar with the anal region, as with any other part of the body, is useful in many ways: It gives us an idea of what we like and don't like; it facilitates communication with partners about sex; and it helps us to get to know our bodies better.

If you're squeamish about looking at or touching yourself down there (and even if you're not), take a bath or shower first so that the area is as clean as you like.

### Don't Be in a Hurry

You'll need a block of uninterrupted time, ideally when you can be alone for a couple of hours. Even if your exploration only lasts twenty minutes, it will be more enjoyable if you don't feel rushed and if you have plenty of time afterward to think about what happened. Rushing is often a way to avoid intimacy and exploration.

### Find a Quiet Place with Some Privacy

Be sure that you won't be startled or interrupted. Do whatever it takes to feel comfortable and in control of your space—lock the door, play some music, disconnect the phone, turn off the doorbell if you can. Dim the lights if you wish. It's important that you feel relaxed and safe.

### Relax

Lying in a comfortable position, take some slow, deep breaths. Breathing is a key to comfortable anal play, as it helps to relax the anus, and relaxation is one of the three essentials to anal erotic pleasure: relaxation, lubrication, and communication.

One technique for increasing your level of relaxation is to work your way up the body, alternately tensing and relaxing various body parts as you inhale and exhale: the toes, ankles, knees, tops of the thighs, pelvis, belly, chest, shoulders, elbows, wrists, fingers, neck, face, forehead. At the end of the sequence, tense all of the parts at once on the inhalation, hold for several seconds, and then collapse completely on the exhalation. You can repeat this part as many times as you wish. Later on, you can share this activity with a partner if you wish. Many people do some form of breath work or stretching, such as yoga, before play. It's a healthy habit to develop, and the preparation will help you to leave the mundane world behind as you enter the erotic one.

## Exploration

Now find a comfortable position where you can stay for a while. Get a hand mirror and some good light. Position yourself so that you can see your butt in the mirror. Take a look at your anus. How does it look? Does it look tense, relaxed, or somewhere in-between? What's the color? Is there much hair around it?

Gently massage the area around the anus—the inner thighs, the butt, the top of the butt around the tail-bone. Notice how your anus responds. Gradually work your way down to the anus and begin to touch it gently. Notice the sensations you feel in your anus and the rest of your body. Don't penetrate the anus, just stick to external touching for now. Stop when you've explored enough. If you wish, you can write down your observations and feelings in a notebook.

You can repeat the above exercise as many times as you like. You may want to combine touching with masturbation and see how that feels.

### Exploring Penetration

It's a good idea to have a bowel movement and to wash the anus before penetrative play. In fact, taking a bath or shower beforehand is an excellent way to relax. You can even do some exploratory touching, if you wish. Normally, there will be only trace amounts of fecal matter left in the rectum after a bowel movement. If you wish, you can rinse your rectum of any residual fecal matter. See Chapter Four, "Hygiene and Diet," for instructions and suggestions.

You can use your bare fingers or slip on form-fitting gloves made of latex or nitrile. (Vinyl gloves tend to be baggy and thus I don't recommend them for any kind of anal play.) It's a good idea to wash your hands with antibacterial soap or dishwashing liquid both before and after play. Your nails should be trimmed and filed so that they're smooth and have no edges or rough spots. You'll also need some lubricant.

Begin with the same kind of preparation and relaxation you chose for the looking and touching exercise.

### Get Greasy

I recommend that you use an oil-based lube if you're playing alone. However, bear in mind that oil-based lubes will destroy latex, which may not be an issue for you in your solo exploration. If your glove or condom starts losing its integrity, though, you'll know why. (In any case, *don't* use an oil-based lube with latex condoms or gloves when playing with a partner!)

Silicone lube is a decent second choice, since it has a consistency similar to "pre-come" (nature's lubricant!) and stays moist for quite a while. However, don't use silicone lube with silicone toys, as it may ruin them— the lube and the silicone toy aren't compatible.

You can find thick, water-based lubes marketed especially for anal play. Water-based lubes tend to dry out and need refreshing with water. If you do choose water-based lube for your exploration, a small plant mister or similar water-filled spray bottle comes in handy for reviving lube. (Recycled

---

**Have Everything You Need at Hand Before You Start**

- Lube.
- Toys.
- Towels (big ones for under your body, and small ones for cleanup later).
- Drinking water, perhaps.
- Plenty of pillows.
- Mirrors can be fun.
- You may want a small flashlight.
- Adequate heat. Make sure you're warm enough—too much heat is better than too little.

Bactine bottles are great for this and also travel well.) However, dealing with this rehydration problem is distracting and can break the flow of play. See Chapter Six, "Latex and Lube," for more information on choosing lubes for anal play.

Don't be afraid to get greasy. One of the wonders of this type of play is the sense of limitless abandon that one can achieve, which is its own form of ecstasy. It's much easier to attain this sense of freedom when you don't have to restrict your body movement because of logistical or aesthetic concerns like grease on the couch. Have enough towels on hand to avoid worrying about staining the sheets or furniture.

## It All Starts with a Finger

Begin massaging your anus with a single lubricated finger. Experiment with different types of motion to see what feels good. Many people like to use a slow, circular motion; others prefer an up-and-down or a back-and-forth motion. You can also try rubbing first on one side of your anus and then the other, pulling outward with a stretching motion. You can use more than one finger at once if you wish. There's no correct way to do this, as long as it doesn't hurt. If something hurts, then stop doing it and rest. Then try doing something else. Just keep breathing deeply, and don't go any faster than is comfortable.

When you feel comfortable, try slipping the tip of your lubricated finger into your anus using slow motions. Find the two sphincters and notice how elastic they are. If it feels good, you can try dipping the finger in further, adding a second finger, or spreading the sensation outward from your sphincters in different directions. It's all up to you.

### Exploring with Toys

Our culture puts a lot of emphasis on intercourse, but it's safer and easier to explore and enjoy anal penetration by starting with fingers and perhaps a small butt toy. A toy designed for anal use is safer than a surrogate such as a cucumber or carrot, which could slip all the way inside you and be difficult or painful to remove. Make sure that any toy you intend to use anally has a base at least an inch wider than the penetrating part.

Anal toys such as dildos, vibrators, and butt plugs should be cleaned and disinfected before use. You may also want to keep them covered with a condom during play. Chapter Seven, "Tools and Toys," comprehensively covers the types of anal toys available today; that's also where you'll find detailed information on cleaning toys. You may skip ahead and read the section on cleaning right away, or save it for later. The important thing to know for now is to keep your toys clean and never to share a toy that hasn't been disinfected.

When you're learning how to use toys, be experimental and don't rush. You'll be more successful with inserting toys if you keep an open, relaxed mind and don't try to impose your own ideas on how things should go. Pay really close attention to your internal and external sphincters. You don't want to cause any tearing or other discomfort that could put a halt to your explorations.

Jack Morin's "biofeedback" exercise is helpful when you're starting your exploration. With this exercise, you simply slip your lubricated finger (or fingers) into your anal canal and describe the current tensed or relaxed state of your internal sphincter. Insert your finger so that you can feel the sphincter and say aloud, "tense, tense" or "relax, relax" as you feel the internal sphincter tensing or relaxing. Increase the number of fingers as you feel comfortable doing so, until you're ready to try inserting the toy. Again, deep, conscious breathing helps to develop body awareness and relaxation. You always want to insert on the exhalation.

Don't insert the toy any more quickly, any further, or for any longer than is comfortable for *you*. If you're using a new plug, for instance, it may be too wide to accommodate initially. Experiment with alternatives such as putting it in a little bit with an in-and-out motion, or even switching to a smaller, narrower, or differently shaped toy. See Chapter Seven to learn how to shop for the right toy.

Sometimes, switching to a different position makes an enormous difference. You'll find a lot of material on different positions for intercourse in Chapter Nine, "Penetration," although you don't need a partner to experiment with positions. In fact, you can skip ahead to Chapter Nine right away if you want some ideas on positions for solo play.

The best way to develop control and capacity is to do your Kegels and breathing exercises consistently (see Chapter Two, "How It Works, and How to Work It").

Don't push too hard on anything that's making you sore. It's far better to let the sphincters do the driving. When the mind and the body are aligned, the toy will be more likely to find its way in.

## Masturbation

Did I mention that it's OK to masturbate in conjunction with all this activity? You probably figured that out, anyhow! Still, I've placed the solo material before the partnered material in this book for a very good reason: The safest and most comfortable way to experiment with anal sex, at least initially, is in solitude. If you want to try any of the things in this book with a partner, it just makes sense to experiment with your own body first. You can never fully appreciate how something feels to your partner if you lack direct experience. Learning to give *yourself* anal pleasure is the very best way to understand what it takes to give your partner the ecstasy he or she desires.

Almost all men masturbate, even if they sometimes feel guilty about it. The man who feels that masturbation is a bad habit, or a sin, is more likely to get it over with as quickly as possible than he is to experiment with or enhance the experience. Many men never experiment with anal masturbation at all. That's sad. If you feel guilty about masturbation or anal pleasure, please ask yourself why you're afraid to feel good about it. If you want to try something on a partner but not on yourself, then ask yourself, why would your partner enjoy it if *you're* afraid to?

Masturbation aside, the main purpose of the exploratory process is to focus on the anal region so that you become more comfortable with its look, its feel, and its sensations. Furthermore, since the outer sphincter of the anus tends to tighten in conjunction with any genital contractions, I recommend saving masturbation to orgasm until *after* you're comfortable with any touching or penetration, especially if you're inserting anything larger than your finger. If your anus gets too tight, you can stop masturbating for a while and go back to the breath work and gentle finger stimulation until it relaxes again. Don't restrict your masturbation to the genitals, either. Some people discover that stimulating other erogenous zones, such as their nipples, enhances their anal experiences. Once again, it pays to keep an open, experimental mind.

*I was playing with a new butt plug. I'd had a friend use it on me a week or so prior to playing with it myself, and we'd had fun with it, but it was just too big and wide to stay put; plus, the base was shallow, so there wasn't much for my sphincter to grab onto. This time, when I was alone, I opened myself up with my fingers, using plenty of grease, and that was pretty successful—soon I was open enough to insert all but my thumb, so I began inserting the plug, in and out, slowly like a dildo or a penis. I took many breaks and didn't rush.*

*It took forty minutes before I was open enough to hold the plug in for any length of time, but, man! Once I felt my butt sucking it in and gripping it, it was paradise. Then I could create resistance by pretending I was pulling it out, and my anus would clamp down on it, and the reverberations throughout my hole were just incredible. This went on for maybe ten or fifteen minutes. It sounds weird, but I really bonded with that toy. Eventually I began jacking off, which led to a shattering orgasm and the hugest ejaculation I'd seen come out of me in months, even though I'd come just twelve hours earlier. I bellowed my guts out! I can't wait to try it again.*

 **Playing with Toys**

> Try a solo run with a butt plug or dildo. Remember to start small, go slowly, and relax. The point isn't to accommodate the biggest butt plug in the toy box, but to experiment with sensation and find out what you like.

# 4

# Hygiene and Diet

## Basic Anal Hygiene

There's no one correct way to do hygiene before anal play. There are *many*, and if you pay attention to your body and its functioning, particularly the digestive system, you'll develop a routine that works for you. What I can offer you here is a set of guidelines that will help you figure out your own preferences.

At a minimum, it's a good idea to bathe or shower after your last bowel movement and before anal play. Your fingernails should be trimmed and clean before any sort of anal hygiene or play.

Wash the anal region with soap and water. You'll feel (and smell) much fresher. Think of it as the gentlemanly thing to do. Some folks find it erotic to do this with a partner, underneath a running shower.

When we start to play, most of us worry a little about finding poop in our rectums, which is a legitimate concern. It can be messy and inconvenient, and perhaps embarrassing if we're with a partner. Understanding how feces move through the lower colon and rectum can help us feel less fearful of this process.

## A Bit of Anatomy, Again

Feces are generally stored in the colon, located above the rectum. When pressure builds up, the colorectal sphincter separating colon from rectum opens up and the feces descend into the rectum. This is what's happening when you get that full feeling that tells you it's time to sit on the toilet—your body wants to expel the waste that has just moved into the rectum. If this happens at a time when it's not convenient to use the toilet, we contract a group of muscles called the pelvic sling and, to a lesser extent, the anal sphincter muscles.

So any poop in the rectum is most likely a vestige from the last bowel movement, or has moved into the rectum and has been withheld from expelling. If there's leftover poop in the rectum after a bowel movement, its presence may be a result of its consistency.

## Step One: Sit and Relax

One secret to having a consistently empty rectum prior to anal play is to develop the habit of going to the toilet as soon as you get that full feeling. Ideally, you'll have your last bowel movement about an hour before sex. (If you're doing a deep rinse or an enema, which are essentially self-administered bowel movements, you'll want to allow *two* hours; there's more on that later in this chapter.)

Sit on the toilet to see if you can expel any feces that are already in your rectum. This makes the whole process easier and less time-consuming. Don't worry if nothing comes out, though; it's just a good idea to check. There's no need to force feces out, either. Just relax, breathe slowly and deeply, and take your time.

In fact, relaxation is the best preparation for cleaning out, just as with any form of anal play. Unless the cleansing process is an integral part of your play with your partner, you'll likely want to do it alone. Anal douching also tends to be somewhat noisy—sploosh!—so if you're nervous about someone overhearing your preparation, try to find a time and place where you can be assured of privacy. You can use many of the same relaxation techniques we covered in the previous chapter: soft lighting, appropriate mood music, and so forth.

### Squatting vs. Sitting

Have you traveled in East Asia? If so, you know that a typical Asian toilet is a hole in the floor (or in the ground); you squat so that your anus is almost as low as your feet. Asians often squat when resting, working, and such; the butt doesn't touch the floor. This is very different from Westerners' resting the butt directly on a chair, or on the ground. Posturally, squatting is the best way of shitting. It allows for more complete elimination. However, squatting on a Western toilet is precarious, and one must be barefoot to do this safely.[1]

### Step Two: Self-Check

You can always check for the presence of feces by inserting a lubricated finger into your rectum. If the thought of this disgusts you, you can use a latex glove or do it in the shower so that you can immediately rinse away any clinging particles.

Although thick, oil-based lubricants such as Vaseline can destroy condoms (and thus are no good for use prior to protected anal intercourse), they can be useful for doing a self-check, as they tend to act as an insulator for anal contact. In other words, they usually cover up any smell or transfer of fecal matter. Wiping off with a dry cloth or paper towel generally results in your finger (or penis, or toy) seeming to be just about perfectly clean. Of course, you should still follow up with hot water and antibacterial soap.

## Step Three: Internal Cleansing

Strictly speaking, internal cleansing—also known as rinsing or douching with an enema bulb or bag or with a shower attachment—isn't necessary for enjoyable, successful anal play. While in this chapter I discuss several options for rinsing the anal cavity, none of them is a necessary preparation for anal sex. Many anal enthusiasts, though, find them desirable. The more deeply you explore anal play—and I use the word "deeply" in the physical as well as the conceptual sense—the more likely it is that this type of preparation will make sense to you.

If you're lucky enough to have an experienced, trusted partner who is willing to help you through your first several experiences with rinsing out, by all means take advantage of the opportunity. If not, don't worry; just follow these step-by-step instructions:

1. Lubricate the anus and nozzle of the enema bag or shower attachment. Use enough lube to permit the nozzle to pass comfortably through the anus and into the rectum.

2. Insert the nozzle. Gently place the tip of the nozzle against the anus and slowly tip it in. Try not to clench at this point. Your anus may be more relaxed and receptive if you push gently as you exhale. You can put yourself in any position that feels comfortable—lying on your side, curled; on your back with

your legs elevated; crouching on all fours; or bending forward while standing. You don't need to insert the nozzle all the way, just far enough to ensure that the water flows into you without spitting out.

3. Let the water flow. Squeeze the bulb, release the clamp, or whatever is appropriate for your nozzled device. Let the water flow into you for as long as it takes you to count to 10—or perhaps 7 for a beginner! The sensation of water rushing into you is strange at first and takes a bit of getting used to. Don't take in any more water than you feel comfortable holding. Note: If you're using a low-capacity bulb syringe or similar device, you may want to take in several batches of water in succession before evacuating.

4. Hold the water. Stop the flow of water into your rectum and hold it in for a few moments. Take a few breaths and allow yourself to feel the fullness.

5. Expel the water. Blot the remaining moisture around your anus when you're done. People who douche more than occasionally sometimes modify or remove the drain plate in their tub or shower to allow any solid matter to flow quickly down the drain—this is a convenience that avoids the need for repeated climbing in and out of the tub. Otherwise, the toilet is fine.

6. Repeat several times or until the water expelled runs clear. Don't overdo it. Two or three repetitions should be fine; more may irritate the delicate lining of your anal canal.

By the way, wanting to pee frequently during the process is normal, since your gut will be absorbing water from your douche and passing it on to the bladder. So pee as often as you like; releasing the bladder makes it easier and more comfortable to clean out.

That's it, basically. Everything else I discuss in this chapter (and there's a lot to talk about, actually) elaborates on this simple routine.

## Three Options for Cleansing

There are three major approaches to cleansing: a quick rinse, a deep rinse, and an erotic enema.

### Quick rinse

The first, most basic approach is a quick rinsing of the rectum for those who just want to feel a bit fresher inside before receptive analingus, anal intercourse, finger play, or butt toy play. Usually a series of three or four shallow rinses is enough to do the trick. Another motive for a light cleansing could be as part of a regular hygiene routine. Some people just like rinsing out their butt in much the same way that some like to gargle with mouthwash—it helps them feel fresh.

> ### Here's What You'll Need
>
> • Lube.
> • Towel for drying off, and possibly paper towels or folded sheets of toilet paper for blotting after each expulsion.
> • Device with nozzle for insertion into the anus (bulb syringe, enema bag, or shower shot), filled with warm to tepid water. Body temperature or slightly warmer water should be about right. Some devices include an inflatable "bardex" attachment to ensure that the hose stays inserted. See Chapter Fourteen, "Resources," for a list of suppliers of enema equipment.
> • You'll also want some way of rinsing off, which is why many people douche in a shower or bathtub.

### Deep rinse

The second approach is a lengthier process as a preparation for more advanced anal play, such as fisting, also known as handballing (see Chapter Ten, "Fisting"), or perhaps for the insertion of larger toys. This kind of preparation is more elaborate and can take up to two hours. A number of approaches can be tried. Some enthusiasts engage in several cleaning sessions over several hours, while others just keep flushing themselves until they're cleaned out, often using progressively larger amounts of water.

This process has several stages. At first, the material you dump will be fairly solid; depending on your diet, it may be large chunks or small nuggets. Generally this material comes from the rectum. As the water reaches into the colon, the second stage will consist of softer, squishier matter that looks more like clay, while the third stage involves the expulsion of brown liquid containing flecks and very small pieces of matter. Usually, the very final stage involves rinsing out the rectum or both rectum and the colon until the expelled water runs clear.

### Erotic enema

The third approach to cleansing isn't necessarily a preparation; rather, it's an erotic, often elaborate, process unto itself. While someone has yet to write the great how-to book on erotic enemas and colonics, *The Enema as an Erotic Art and Its History,* by David Barton-Jay, is an excellent start.[2] If you're interested in the erotic potential of the enema, I recommend that you track down a copy of this quirky and hard-to-find book. Bear in mind, however, that some folks find enemas to be a major turn-off, often because of trauma related to enforced enema-taking when they were children. (It used to be a fairly common method for treating constipation.) If this is the case for you or your partner, I recommend that you proceed carefully, patiently, and with plenty of communication. You may even want to enlist the help of a sympathetic therapist to work through any difficulties.

## How Much Rinsing Is Enough?

There's no absolutely right answer because each of us is unique, temperamentally and anatomically. Also, as you can see above, it depends on your intent. Basically, though, you rinse until the water runs clean out of the rectum. What you have in your gut on a particular day varies widely, as does your level of stress and numerous other factors. Thus, on one occasion, cleaning out may be quick and easy for you, while on another, the identical procedure may not be as effective. The large intestine has a number of twists and turns, and its exact position, size, and shape varies from person to person. So the cleaning-out process is unique for each of us, and in time, novices will develop their own techniques for efficient cleansing.

I advise that you be cautious and go slowly when you're first experimenting with douching, as too much rinsing can irritate your rectum and curtail your play. Your butt will simply shut down if you overdo anything. Douching does rinse away some of the protective mucosal lining, which is why some experts recommend, as a precaution, that you allow about two hours after the last rinse for the rectum to reline itself before intercourse.

Will regular douching cause you to lose your ability to evacuate normally? Or eventually make you incontinent? No. It's certainly possible to irritate the colon through overuse of enemas. However, if you use common sense, you won't hurt yourself. The muscles of the anus are highly elastic, and your colon and rectum operate in the same fashion whether or not you're giving yourself enemas. In fact, there is support for the use of an enema in many holistic health practices. For example, the yogic tradition encourages developing the ability to use the anal sphincter to suck water into the rectum for a ritual rinse.

Most folks not into enemas, fisting, or large toys play with the last six inches of the large intestine—the anal sphincters and the rectum. Rinsing beyond that pushes water into the colon, which may trigger expulsion of additional, usually looser, fecal matter, a process that can be hard to curtail once you've started it. You may end up spending more time rinsing than playing before you feel clean!

## Three Devices for Rinsing

Three rinsing tools are in common use: the enema kit, the shower diverter, and the bulb syringe. The basic premise behind each of these tools is the same; each uses water pressure to evacuate feces. Many people, even authorities on anal sex, mention enema bags in the same breath with shower diverters; some don't even mention shower diverters at all, perhaps because they don't know about them. Yet once you overcome the oddity of feeling a liquid enter your butt, the experiences are very different.

### Enema Kits

Commercial enema kits (the kind you buy in a drugstore) usually come in a cardboard box and consist of a one- or two-quart rubber bag with a hose attached; a plastic hook to hang the bag; two different nozzles (either of which can be used for anal douching); and a stopper to convert the bag to use as a hot-water bottle. Some disposable kits contain a cheaper, clear plastic bag and hose.

Specialty suppliers catering to enema enthusiasts carry a wide array of unique enema devices, and they're coming up with new items all the time. Among the items I've seen in the past few years is a large-capacity, hanging

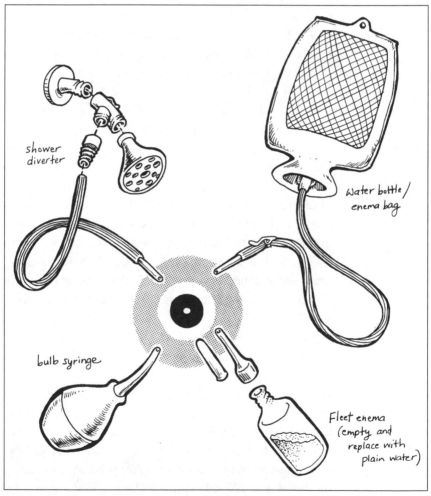

shower diverter

Water bottle / enema bag

bulb syringe

Fleet enema (empty and replace with plain water)

**Illustration # 4: Enema Equipment**

Plexiglas cylinder with enough valves and hoses to make Dr. Frankenstein's lab seem tame. Larger-capacity rubber bags and open-top bags are popular with enema fetishists, too. Some suppliers are listed in the Resources.

Fill the bag or bottle with water. Hang it from a hook placed higher than the body (but no more than 18 inches). If the hose barely reaches your anus, the bag is too high. If more than half of it extends below your anus, it's too low. Release the hose clamp and let the water run briefly to expel any cramp-causing air that remains in the system. Lightly lubricate the anus and the nozzle (taking care not to clog the nozzle), insert the nozzle into the rectum, and release the bag's contents. Use the hose clamp as necessary to control the flow of liquid.

Once you're as full as you wish to be (usually after about 10 seconds), stop the flow and release the liquid into the toilet or down the drain. Alternately, you can hold it for a while and then release it. (Some folks find retaining the liquid for as long as possible to be an erotic activity in itself.) Some folks like to massage the gut as they hold the liquid, starting at the sternum, pressing and releasing the abdomen, gradually working their way down to the pubic bone and then releasing the liquid.

## POSITION AND LOCATION FOR ENEMAS

There's no hard and fast rule concerning position or location for receiving an enema. You can receive an enema wherever it feels comfortable for you: in bed (lay some towels underneath you, in case of seepage), in the bathtub, over the toilet, or in the shower. Experiment to find what feels most comfortable for you. Some folks like squatting over a drain or toilet; others prefer being on their back; still others like to be on their knees, butt in the air, while others favor lying on the left side, right leg drawn over the left (the standard "hospital" position). Many find that lying down helps the water move higher into the gut and thus facilitates evacuation. A combination of lying and standing works best for some. I have even known people who like to do knee bends or exaggerated marching-in-place motions, bringing each knee to the opposite side of the chest. Some people press and massage their belly to encourage complete elimination.

If you're prone to gas problems, you can lie on your back with your feet raised so that your butt is higher than your intestines. This position allows the water to work its way behind the gas bubbles so that the water pushes the bubbles out when you expel it. There are additional suggestions for dealing with gas in the section on diet, below.

## SOME TIPS FOR USING ENEMA BAGS

Filling the bag completely helps to avoid air, which causes cramping. Remember to let a bit of the water flow out of the nozzle before inserting it. This will push out any air that might be in the system. Besides giving you cramps, air can block the water from getting high enough to clean you out. Since air floats on water, standing while taking water causes any air present to move higher into the gut. This is why some people prefer taking an enema while lying down.

Deep, relaxed breaths will help the liquid flow into you. A tight anus will usually repel a shallow nozzle and create a watery mess as the contents of the bag spray across your bathroom. Don't take in any more water than you feel comfortable with.

The optimal temperature for enema water is roughly body temperature. Hot water causes you to expel more quickly and may be uncomfortable.

You can vary the height of the bag by using a wire hanger. And be sure to weight-test any curtain rod, towel rack, picture hanger, coat hook, or other likely spot for dangling the bag *before* you attempt to use it to hang your enema bag.

## ADDING OTHER INGREDIENTS TO AN ENEMA

Some people like to add various substances to the water. You shouldn't add anything to your enema until you can clean out with no problems. Then, if you want to add something, start slowly and use it sparingly, and never change in mid-session (for instance, from one kind of soap to another). This is the best way to determine what works and what doesn't. Pay close attention to your body for several days afterward to check for after-effects.

Some sources recommend a quarter-teaspoon of table salt per quart of water to replace the sodium your body sheds during an enema. One source suggests that the water should taste about as salty as tears.[3] (However, drinking Gatorade does pretty much the same thing.) In *The Hand Book,* Bert Herrman suggests adding some baking soda to the next-to-last rinse for a soothing effect; he also states that a final rinse of somewhat cooler water may soothe the system as well.[4]

While it's wise to avoid harsh soaps, some people enjoy a small amount of liquid castile soap mixed into the rinse. Soap acts as an irritant that induces fecal matter to expel, but it also tends to wash away the protective mucosal lining. Again, don't overdo it.

Castor oil is given orally as an irritant laxative. It will evacuate you very quickly but can cause cramping and may leave your rectum too irritated to play. I have also heard of douching with olive oil, vegetable oil, or mineral oil. Six ounces is the usual hospital dose of mineral oil for evacuating hard stool in the rectum. This is certainly not enough to do the job you want, it's messy to clean up, and it will probably leave an oily residue in your toilet or drain. Using larger quantities may even block the rectum from its natural digestive function of absorbing vitamins, minerals, and other nutrients. Self-inducing malnutrition is not a great idea!

Some people like to douche with wine or other forms of alcohol. Raw alcohol should never be given as an enema, as it can damage you. The body processes alcohol through the liver, so consuming it rectally circumvents this process. Alcohol is a cellular poison that burns internal tissue. The mucosa absorbs the alcohol even more quickly than the stomach does when sipped, which means that you'll get really drunk really fast and perhaps poison yourself.

> **Mineral Oil**
>
> Plain old mineral oil does have its place in sex play—if you're a man who likes oilier lubes for jacking off. Mineral oil works great, is widely available at drugstores and warehouse stories such as Costco, and is very inexpensive— a little goes a long way. Also, it's flavorless, so if your partner wants to go down on you after you've been jacking off, it's pretty inoffensive. In my experience, it seems fine to use a small amount for anal play; you can also use a bit to cut thicker, oil-based lubes such as Shaft or Crisco. Finally, mineral oil makes an impromptu massage oil when nothing more specialized is available.

Experiencing a light buzz by putting a couple of teaspoons of wine in a regular enema is probably OK for most people, but if you try this, please be careful and don't overdo it. Always give your body at least a week to recover before doing this again.

**Shower Diverters**

A shower diverter is a piece of steel, brass, or plastic hardware that you insert between the wall pipe and the shower head. As its name suggests, you use a switch to divert the flowing water from the shower head into the douche hose.

"Shower shot" kits—complete with diverter, hose, and in some cases a metal or plastic nozzle—are available from the suppliers listed in Chapter Fourteen, "Resources." The cost for a kit with a nozzle is usually about $60. Alternately, you can make your own kit, which has several advantages over either the enema-bag or the shower kit technique (including a much lower price and a more comfortable alternative to the water-pressure method of evacuation). See "Do-It-Yourself Internal Cleansing Device," below.

If you're purchasing a shower diverter setup, I recommend that you buy metal rather than plastic pieces, as too much pressure causes the plastic to crack readily, and plastic threads strip more easily than durable metal.

SOME TIPS FOR USING SHOWER DIVERTERS

Make sure that any other appliance that draws on the same water source as your shower is turned off during your douche. Laundry machines, dishwashers, and even toilets can cause sudden fluctuations in the water temperature or volume.

You want the water temperature to be about the same as your body temperature, or a little cooler. Some showers, particularly in buildings with older plumbing, can take a while before the temperature stabilizes.

Some tubs are set up so that the shower will only run if there's sufficient pressure to keep the shower stem in the "up" position. If this is the case, I recommend an enema bag or anal spike instead. If you decide to use a shower diverter anyhow, please be extra careful about putting a high-pressure jet of water into your rectum.

Many folks like to use a 9-to-1 water and bleach solution to clean their nozzles. Be aware, however, that some metal nozzles will corrode when left in chlorine bleach. So don't leave metal nozzles overnight in a bleach solution. If possible, get an anodized or stainless nozzle. Some of these nozzles come in a very attractive black.

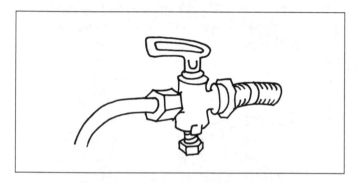

**Illustration # 5: Volume Control Valve**

DO-IT-YOURSELF INTERNAL CLEANSING DEVICE

Commercially available "shower shot" setups consist of a six-foot vinyl hose wrapped in metal coil plus a "silver bullet" attachment made of aluminum or plastic. It will probably cost you around $60. The diverter goes between the wall pipe and the shower head. The flat end of the hose threads into the open half of the diverter.

If your shower head doesn't screw off, or if it's is not readily apparent how to get the diverter between the head and the wall pipe, have a plumber check this out for you. (If you're shy, just say that you are trying to hook up a hand-held shower attachment.)

With a little creativity, you can create your own "shower shot" for much less than the ready-made device. It will be more versatile and do a more reli-

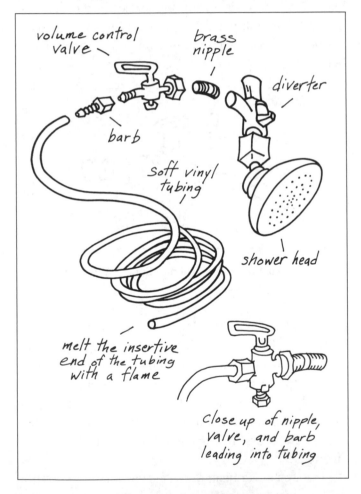

**Illustration # 6: Do-It-Yourself Device**

able and accurate job of cleaning. The reason is that shower shots and enema bags depend on water pressure to clean you out—water is fairly heavy, and when enough water accumulates in your rectum (or possibly your colon), it creates pressure on your sphincters to flush it out. This is a hit-and-miss procedure. It is easy to clean higher or lower than one wants. The system I am about to describe uses very little water pressure and increases the odds of getting the cleansing one wants.

For the do-it-yourself kit, you'll need a volume-control valve and a long piece of soft plastic tubing. Insert the plastic tubing into your butt exactly as far as you want. If you want to be able to take a certain toy, say a six-inch dildo, you need to insert the tubing into your butt six inches. Since you don't need to clean any higher than that, you can use a very low volume of water to rinse out any residual fecal matter.

It may sound a bit extreme to feed a plastic hose up your butt, but two essential steps allow this to work for you. The first is that you must melt the edges of the tubing over a gas flame before using it for the first time. This smoothes the edges. (*Never* insert a sharp edge into any body orifice.)

The second is to use comfortably warm water, because the warmth of the running water softens the plastic. I almost never recommend buying cheap where your comfort and pleasure are concerned, but this is an exception. You need to get the cheaper, *thin* plastic tubing, not the thick kind. Get an eight-foot length, rather than the standard six-foot length that comes with most commercial shower-shot setups. This gives you increased mobility, plus the extra length you'll want for feeding the hose into your rectum.

*Slowly* feed the hose through your anal sphincters, as far as you wish to go into the rectum, or, for experienced players, past the sigmoid colon. Let the water run *slowly* into you until it expels.

## Enemas vs. Shower Diverters

Enemas: Using a bag (also called a "fountain syringe") is somewhat safer than the shower diverter method because there's no chance of sudden fluctuation in water volume or temperature as it flows through a tap. Another advantage is that you can add other ingredients to the water in an enema bag. Also, enema kits are widely available at drugstores, whereas shower diverters can be harder to track down. (Your best bet is a well-equipped hardware store or a fetish supplier.) Diverters also require installation, whereas an enema bag comes ready-to-use. And finally, while you can take an enema bag with you anywhere, hooking up a shower diverter when you travel is usually impractical.

Shower diverters: In case the chief advantage isn't perfectly obvious: no refilling. Having a stream of water ready to serve you for as long as you wish is a tremendous convenience. Plus, some people prefer the feeling of a smooth tube or hose pressing against their anus to the more invasive insertion of the hard plastic enema nozzle. Shower diverters also get the job done more quickly than enema bags because of the higher level of water pressure. You can also adjust the water pressure, whereas an enema bag's pressure is either on or off. (Some specialized enema setups contain flow-control valves, but these are pricey toys sold nowadays by specialty dealers to enema enthusiasts. See Chapter Fourteen, "Resources," for a list of dealers.)

### Bulb Syringes and Related Devices

I should mention one other item in common use: the bulb syringe, a variant of which is called the "anal spike." (Don't worry; it sounds painful, but it's not!) Typically, this is an eight-ounce bulb with a hard plastic nozzle or spike similar to the smaller one that comes with most enema kits. You lubricate and insert the spike into the rectum, then squirt the bulb's water into your rectum, and finally expel it. You may be able to find this device at a drugstore; otherwise, many specialty stores and suppliers catering to fetishists stock it.

An anal spike can be a handy travel companion, as one can usually be tucked into a toilet kit. While some people find that the eight-ounce size is sufficient for their douching needs, others will want the quart-sized capacity of the standard enema bag.

In the same vein, you can buy a commercial preparation such as Fleet, dump the contents of the bottle, and refill with water. Don't use the liquid, as it can irritate the lining of your rectum. Sitting in a tub filled with warm water can work well in conjunction with the bulb syringe. Fill and squeeze the bulb into your rectal cavity several times while seated in the tub, until you feel "full." Wait a few minutes, then sit on the toilet and expel the contents. Repeat the process several times until your bowels expel clean water.

## Kamikaze Cleaning

No one can control all of the conditions and contingencies of his daily life, and there are times when you might decide to have anal sex but lack the time, inclination, or facilities for a relaxed cleaning process. While I don't recommend the following techniques, they are nonetheless real-world solutions that people use when they want to play immediately and must make do with what's available. Since fecal matter can be abrasive to the rectal lining during anal sex, doing something to eliminate residual feces is certainly better than doing nothing, which could end up creating discomfort during play and possibly tear your anal passage.

### Toilet method

You can use lube and a latex glove with this method, or simply a lubricated condom wrapped around your bare finger. If you don't mind contacting fecal matter with your index finger, you can use it unsheathed to lubricate the anus using water-based lube or whatever else is at hand—spit, soap, shaving cream, and so on—although lube intended for sex won't irritate your anus or rectal lining the way that soapy liquids and creams might. Still, if it's a choice between oil-based lube and soap, at least soap won't break condoms, the way oil-based lube might. And again, there's always spit.

Work your finger into the rectum, opening the folds slowly as you go until your finger can't go any further. Slowly and methodically feel around for debris. If you don't find anything, then you've done a good check and you're ready to rock and roll. Otherwise, scoop out any residual feces you contact, dropping it into the bowl or wiping it onto toilet paper. Pull out slowly—if you go too quickly, you risk leaving fecal matter behind. Repeat until you're content that the outermost several inches are clear.

Wipe—if possible, with a damp cloth—and if you didn't use a glove or condom, wash your hands and under the nails thoroughly with soap, preferably an antibacterial liquid such as Dial. Rinse and dry thoroughly. Then be sure to use a condom with any penile penetration.

### Bottle method

Bottled water or soda can be used as an instant douche. Lubricate the anus well before inserting the mouth of the bottle. Let the contents drain slowly into your rectum. A plastic bottle is better, as it's non-breakable and can be squeezed as you would a bulb syringe to ensure maximum effectiveness. Hold as long or as briefly as you wish, and expel. If possible, allow at least 10 to 15 minutes before play to be sure that all of the liquid has drained out.

## Shaving

Like taking an enema, shaving the anal region (or any other body hair) is a hygiene activity that many people find erotic. The main requirements are shaving cream, a good razor, a steady hand, and a heaping helping of trust. Lots of folks who think that getting fucked anally is just dandy have never realized how intimate and vulnerable allowing someone to shave them can be.

Everyone has hair around the asshole. Trimming the hair or shaving it off entirely can make anal penetration easier and more fun—after all, few things bring tears to a hairy-assed tough guy's eyes more quickly than having his butt hairs yanked. Trimming or shaving the hairs has the added bonus of preventing "dingleberries"—those small clumps of fecal matter that cling to butt hair even after wiping. And a smooth, hairless hole is thrilling for some. There may be no better way to more effectively reduce your partner to a quivering little boy or girl than to shave the hair around his or her hole.

If you trim rather than shave, use a pair of manicure scissors or other small, easy to control shears, and leave about a quarter inch of hair to avoid stubble. You can train yourself to shave your own anal region without cutting yourself. Squatting works best since it gives you the greatest access. Some people like to use a small mirror, but this isn't essential if you are careful. Be very gentle with yourself until you've practiced the strokes enough times to be confident that you won't cut yourself. If you have a lot of hair to shave off, you can do it over the course of several showers, taking off a bit more each time. Squatting can be exhausting, so it's best not to do this for a prolonged length of time. You're more likely to cut yourself when tired or uncomfortable.

By the way, don't attempt this with a cheap, disposable razor. It's worth the extra money to use a razor with a flexible, replaceable head, such as the Trac II or Mach III. And don't *ever* use a blade that's been used by anyone else—it may contain bacteria and other germs from contact with that person's blood or from sitting in a moist environment.

I recommend using a manual razor and a light coating of non-irritating shaving cream or soap, rather than an electric razor. Using an electric razor is more likely to lead to snagged or ingrown hairs. By using a manual razor during a shower, it is relatively easy to control the consistency of the cream or to rinse off any excess cream.

Some men and women trim or shave the perineal region, too, and many folks shave some or all of the hair in their genital region. Removing any body hair has consequences—if you don't keep trimming or shaving it, it often causes itchiness as it grows back. You can use a soothing lotion on the area if this is a problem. And don't shave the anogenital region less than a few hours before sex—the tiny nicks and cuts in the skin are an ideal point of entry for viruses (such as HIV) and other germs.

## Notes on Diet

Your diet has an important effect on your ability to enjoy receiving anal play. Much of what I suggest in this section applies primarily to preparation for fisting, but the general principles are useful to anyone interested in any level of anal play.

Many of us don't include adequate fiber in our diet. Fiber promotes soft, well-formed, moist, and bulky stools. Your rectal reflex is triggered more easily with a high-fiber diet, and such a diet has the added advantage of enabling you to relax your internal sphincter muscle more readily. The best sources of fiber are whole grains, beans, peas, nuts, vegetables, and fibrous fresh fruits, such as bananas and apples. Nuts are a good fiber source if you're not planning any anal play in the immediate future; more on this in a moment. Alternately, you can try adding a dose of Metamucil or another fiber supplement to your diet every day.

While for many of us it's neither possible nor practical to continuously control our day-to-day food intake, ideally you'd begin your preparation by watching your diet a few days before playing. Avoid eating berries containing small seeds (including jams and preserves) starting thirty-six to forty-eight hours before play. The abrasive seeds can hide in the folds of the rectum and scratch delicate tissue during play. For the same reason, nuts are also best avoided, as well as poppy, sesame, and other seeds (including those in bread).

During the last eighteen to twenty-four hours prior to anal sex, one source recommends avoiding consuming foods that bind, such as dairy products, meats, and highly processed foods.[5] However, another recommends that you eat little, but that what you do eat be slow to digest, such as eggs and dairy products.[6] I suggest that you experiment to find what's most compatible with your particular system. Increase your intake of vegetables and fruits. Some players recommend bananas to increase your potassium level, as a potassium deficiency can cause dizziness, tremors, and other problems, particularly during heavy play.

On the day you plan to play, eat lightly. It takes about twelve hours for food to enter the large intestine, and about twelve more to leave. So ideally, you'd cut back on heavy food starting about twelve hours before you cleanse. A hot drink about fifteen minutes before play can aid in flushing the system and may help you to relax.

Some people like to eat yogurt or take acidophilus capsules to help the intestine restore its balance of "good bugs" —microorganisms that aid in food digestion and waste elimination but that get rinsed away during douching.

## Avoiding and Dealing with Gas

Much of the discomfort that people report from douching or other anal penetration comes from trapped gas bubbles. Gas makes it difficult or even impossible to clean out completely. Try changing your diet if it contains a lot of fructose, or if you are lactose-intolerant and consume dairy products, or if you have suddenly increased your fiber intake.

Over-the-counter products like Beano can help relieve gas pressure, as can the more common range of overeating remedies such as Di-Gel, Alka-Seltzer, Pepto-Bismol, Rolaids, and the rest. I keep a supply of Zantac (ranitidine) handy. And if there's nothing else around, you can always drink a dose of baking soda dissolved in warm water every twenty to thirty minutes until the discomfort has passed.

You can also try lying on your side during ass play (some say that the left side is best), or in the pregnancy antigas position: Get on your knees and lean forward until you're in a prone position, remaining on your knees with your butt in the air and your chest resting on the bed or floor. Rest your head on your hands and keep your butt in the air (gas rises).

Massage can also help. Try massaging your stomach while taking deep, slow breaths to push the gas toward the rectum, relax the anal sphincters, and allow the gas to pass. Some folks find it relaxing to reach back and gently massage the area just underneath the tailbone, where the cleft between the cheeks begins. That's because this helps to relax the external sphincter, which is where we hold a lot of tension when we're trying not to pass gas.

Passing gas with a partner present is embarrassing for most of us. It just happens sometimes, and if you're interested in anal sex, the problem will surface (ahem!) at some point. If you feel a gas wave coming on, and you want to spare your partner—and yourself—the indignity, you can excuse yourself. However, it's probably best just to accept this as a fact of anal sex.

Some people, such as HIV-positive folks on medications, have frequent diarrhea that can get in the way of anal play. If this poses a problem for you, you can try a few things. Experiment with eliminating spicy foods from your diet, as these can irritate the bowel and trigger diarrhea. I have also heard that bananas tend to solidify the feces. You can also take Imodium, Lomitil, or other remedies that stop the flow of diarrhea. Imodium is usually effective for about twenty-four hours after taking it. Finally, if you're HIV-positive, time your medications to avoid diarrhea—that is, don't take them right before sex.

NOTES

1. Correspondence with Tortuga Bi Liberty, San Francisco, December 2001.

2. David Barton-Jay, *The Enema as an Erotic Art and Its History* (The David Barton-Jay Projects, P.O. Box 1235, Brattleboro, VT 05302, 1996).

3. www.pigmedia.com/health.htm

4. Bert Herrman, Trust: *The Hand Book (A Guide to the Sensual and Spiritual Art of Handballing)*, (Alamo Square Press, 1991), p. 36.

5. Sexuality.org, "Handballing Guide," www.sexuality.org/l/sex/handball.html

6. Sexuality.org, "Handballing FAQ," www.sexuality.org/l/incoming/aanal.html

# Communication

While most interpersonal communication is nonverbal, open discussion about anal sex before, during, and after sex increases the likelihood that you and your partner will have a successful and enjoyable experience you'll want to repeat.

If you're in a partnered relationship or seeing someone regularly, it will be easier for you to bring up the possibility of anal sex if your relationship already includes open and relaxed discussions about sex. If you're not yet comfortable talking about sex with your partner, start by discussing the sex you are *already* having together before you bring up the idea of trying something new. You can use this nonthreatening four-step DESC process:[1]

- Describe the current situation nonjudgmentally. For example: "I've really been enjoying our lovemaking, but I have a hard time talking about sex, and I'd like to change that."
- Express your feelings about this situation. "When we don't share our likes and dislikes about something that's so important, I don't feel as close to you as I'd like to."
- Specify the changes you wish. "So I would really like it if we could discuss sex more openly."
- Spell out the consequences of this change—taking care to emphasize the positive ones that will result from the behavior change, rather than the negative ones for noncompliance. "Talking about sex, especially about what feels good, and maybe even about some new things, could make our lovemaking even better."

In any case, it's wise to start talking about sex, anal or otherwise, in a nonsexual setting rather than right before you have sex. Because of the anal taboo, this is a difficult subject for many of us to broach. Your partner may even have thought of it himself or herself but could be having a hard time bringing it up. There's also a chance that he or she will be turned off or even horrified when you mention anal sex. In that case, you can give your partner a dozen roses along with a copy of this book!

You can try the indirect approach and see how your partner reacts. Bring up anal sex in a general way, perhaps a bit playfully, to test his or her reaction. That should cue you as to how to proceed. If you enjoy sharing print or video pornography, try bringing home some material that includes anal pleasure. Not all porn is created equal, so if possible, prescreen it before sharing with your partner. You can find many reputable sources for anal erotica and instructional material in Chapter Fourteen, "Resources." Discussing any erotic or instructional material after experiencing it together is an important precursor to experimenting with anal sex yourselves, since this is the best time to address any fears or concerns regarding play. You can also look at sex toy catalogs or browse online sex toy catalogs or images of anal sex. Another possibility is to talk about your own anal explorations— or even masturbate for your partner, incorporating anal play.

In any event, *do not* try anal sex with your partner for the first time without discussing it beforehand. Initial experiences with penetration, in particular, can be challenging enough without the added element of surprise. Trying to "trick" your lover into anal sex or going at it too aggressively may upset them so much that you never get the chance to try it a second time.

> ### Especially for the Novice
>
> It's essential to be up-front about your level of experience. If you're a novice or relatively new to anal intimacy, your partner needs to know that. Anal play is one activity that you simply should not fake your way through. Countless men and women have been turned off to anal sex permanently because of a few initial negative experiences.
>
> The first and most essential ingredient for anal intimacy is desire. For ability to increase, desire must increase first. In many cases, though, our desire to try something new is overshadowed by our fear of it, and anal sex is no exception. While fear can be a powerful aphrodisiac in some erotic settings, it usually gets in the way of our acting on our desire, and it certainly gets in the way of anal sex, since a fearful butthole is a closed, tense butthole.

## Togetherness

*The best part of anal sex? Being with somebody with whom I'm emotionally close enough to do it. If I were to qualify something as "best," it wouldn't necessarily be the physical sensations, but the fact that I'm with someone with whom I can share that.*

When you take the time and effort to discuss your desires and fears with your partner, you're more likely to have pleasurable experiences that you will want to repeat. Some topics for discussion include:

- Your wants
- Your limits and ground rules
- Your past experiences—what worked or didn't work for you
- Childhood memories of prevailing attitudes toward anal sex, jokes you've heard about it, how you learned about it
- Your fantasies

## Your Right to Say No

*I was raped. It took years to process that. I shut down, and all kinds of stuff happened without my understanding it. My subconscious was basically taking care of me, but it didn't seem like it at the time. And it's been hard to come back. I've been more cautious, which is good. But some of it really does get in my way. The best thing I did, many years later, when I realized it was an issue, was to write it down and change the ending of the story. I did several versions—one where I threw him out the window and became a spokesperson for rape victims, and another one where he turned into a really sweet person and stopped and said, "We should go slower," and we lived happily ever after. I found it to be very, very powerful.*

It bears repeating that anal sex does *not* have to hurt—not ever. Even if you surrender your power to a partner in an S/M or other "scene" involving power exchange, ultimately you're always in charge of your own pleasure.

And even in an S/M scene, you should reserve the right to say no to anything that you feel is dangerous, excessively painful, or simply "going faster than your turn-on." And since no partner is a mind-reader, no top is going to know what *does* turn you on unless you tell them so. (We'll cover S/M and related play at greater length in Chapter Eleven, "Extreme Sex: S/M, Gender Play, Fetishes, Piss Play, and Scat Play.")

It's wrong to allow yourself to be pressured into a sexual encounter with anyone, ever. Sexual union that isn't wholly desired by both parties is hollow, bereft of

### Safewords

Some people, particularly in the early stages of exploring new forms of sexual play, like to use safewords.

A safeword is a word that the partners have mutually agreed on to stop or slow the action. Of course, you can just say "stop" or "slower," but sometimes, in the heat of passion, the meaning of these common words can become blurred, muted, or otherwise distorted. A well-established convention in the S/M world is to use judiciously the traffic light colors "red" and "yellow." In any case, though, a loud, clear "STOP" means "stop what you're doing," unless you've agreed otherwise (as in a "consensual nonconsensual" S/M scene—more on this in Chapter Eleven.)

real intimacy, and ultimately damaging to the relationship. Even if you spend a year and a day being the world's biggest butt-slut, playing daily with the endless variations on anal sex, you have every right to declare on day 367 that you are over it. Sexual behavior is fluid over time. Frequency and interest both change. And anal sex is no exception.

Don't feel obligated to explain your sexual rhythms to anyone. Sex, or abstinence from sex, or refraining from a particular kind of sex, never needs to be justified. Part of the work involved in a committed relationship, however, involves frank discussion regarding your current state of sexual affairs. If you have continued difficulty talking about a particular aspect of your relationship, such as its sexual dynamic, seeing a couples counselor is an option worth considering.

## Setting the Scene

Sufficient preparation for anal sex frequently affects what occurs during the act itself. Some simple act, such as locking the door, drawing the blinds, or sharing a glass of water or wine, can be very powerful symbolically as a way to draw the veil between the mundane world and the erotic world you're about to enter.

- Privacy. Lock the door, disconnect the phone, turn off the pager, draw the blinds. Do whatever it takes to ensure that you won't be jarred in the midst of play.
- Mood lighting. Lights should be low and indirect, but not so dim that you can't easily see your partner's face or anything that you may be using in your play, like lube or toys. Lighting with warm colors, such as red or amber, helps create the desired

mood. Alternately, you can drape a colored scarf, handkerchief, or thin towel over a lampshade as long as it doesn't create a fire hazard.

- Music. Your choice of background music can heavily impact your experience. You don't want anything so loud that you can't hear each other. Talking about what feels good and listening to the other person's breathing are two important cues when you're having any kind of sex, but even more so with anal sex because the moment-to-moment feedback is so important.

- Supplies. In addition to the obvious tools and toys (lube, condoms, gloves, sex toys—all covered in detail in the next two chapters), have plenty of pillows and towels available. Have something to drink close at hand.

- Take lots of time. You don't want to attempt anal sex when you're feeling rushed. Rushing tends to make real communication difficult, and communication is one of the most important elements of anal penetration (along with patience and lots of lube!).

## Connectedness

If you've discussed trying anal sex with your partner, and even if things have gone swimmingly in your conversation, he or she may still develop a case of "wedding-night jitters." If your partner expresses fear or hesitation about trying anal sex, you can reassure them that you don't want to hurt or upset them and that they can stop or rest if anything you're doing gets uncomfortable. Explain that there are a lot of things you can do anally besides intercourse and that, while penetration may be an option for later, you want to ease into anal play by just trying a few things.

You can hug your partner and assure them that you want this to be as much fun for them as for you. Many of us associate anal sex with violence or force, even subconsciously. So touching your partner in a warm and comforting way as a prelude to anal sex can reassure them that this won't be the case with you.

During any kind of anal play, it's important to check in with your partner periodically, especially when trying anything new. "Is this OK with you?" and "How does that feel?" are two of the most important—and sexiest—questions you can ever ask your partner. You don't need to repeat the questions so often that they become annoying; a periodic check-in is enough. You can even phrase your check-ins in a sexy way: "You like feeling that up there, don't you?" or "Does your butt want some more of that?" And, of course, you can often get much more information just by watching your partner's reactions. But if they're not giving you verbal or physical clues, by all means ask!

Establishing eye contact and "ear contact" are crucial to establishing the kind of deep connection described above. Most people require the moment-to-moment feedback that comes from a constant connection. Presence and timing are important. You should be able to hear the other person's breathing. Tops shouldn't be afraid to ask lots of questions, particularly in the initial stages. Eye contact is vital to draw the other person into your mind-space. Just take your time and do whatever it takes for the two of you to be in sync.

## Emotional Boundaries

Intense sex can dredge up painful emotions that we've been unaware of or have suppressed. The beauty of this phenomenon is that it offers us an opportunity to start to heal the anger, fear, sadness, grief, jealousy, or whatever else comes up. If you can look at the emotion as just what it is—an emotion that is a *reflection* of your reality rather than the thing itself—you can begin letting go of it so that it no longer has so much power over you. Having a partner who has earned your trust can make this process even easier. Sometimes just having someone to talk to can help us resolve our issues more quickly than we could alone. At other times, though, it's best to acknowledge when we're overwhelmed, and continue the discussion when we feel calm and less threatened.

## Control

In sex play, control over the scene should almost always lie with the receptive partner.[2] If you're the receptive partner in a play session, ultimately you orchestrate the speed, the rhythm, the angle, and the duration. You must be aware of your body's sensations and limitations; this is where your experiences with self-exploration can pay off. A good top (or top-in-training) will stop when the bottom tells him to. Don't worry about looking stupid or inadequate. Neither of you should be afraid to talk or ask questions. Whether you are the "doer" or the "do-ee," you're responsible for communicating your anal erotic desires to your partner.

## Sexual Competition

One issue that comes up for many of us, particularly for gay and bisexual men, is competition. We live in a culture where men are encouraged to compete with one another for status. And as much as we might wish to be, gay and bisexual men aren't exempt from the effects of this cultural conditioning—in fact, in the gay community, such conditioning often plays out as sexual competitiveness. There's probably even a biological basis for it—males of many species strut, posture, and sport the brighter colors of the two genders.[3] Whether it's the quest for the hunkiest body, the biggest dick, the handsomest face, or the most voracious bottom, any time you find yourself comparing yourself with others in terms of sexual attractiveness or prowess, you're manifesting this competitive behavior.

Although such behavior is natural, too much emphasis on externals can stand in the way of communication and intimacy. With receptive anal sex, there's the fear that if we express discomfort, our partner will think we're whining and start looking for someone more "playful"—a fear that all too often translates into reality. The irony is that if you feel you have to numb yourself mentally, emotionally, or chemically to please a partner, then you're losing the very intimacy that you sought with him or her in the first place. If this is the case, then you need to discuss this with your partner. If this is a non-negotiable point, then it's time for you to seek couples counseling or find a different partner.

However, this issue is far from unique to gay men. In The Ultimate Guide to Anal Sex for Women, Tristan Taormino urges women, "Don't have anal sex because you think it's what your partner wants. Or because your partner is pressuring you to do it. Or because you're afraid that you won't be a desirable lover if you don't do it. Take responsibility for your erotic likes and dislikes—figure out what they are and then communicate them to your partner."[4]

The point is this: While competitiveness has its purpose and place, ultimately it's not in your best interest to compare your sexual prowess with others. This sets up an unhealthy dynamic where you depend on others for your sense of sexual self-worth. And every one of us deserves better than that.

## Discussing Safer Sex and Degree-of-Risk Issues

You should discuss safer sex and degree-of-risk issues with any new partner before you start having sex, preferably in a nonsexual setting. While I can't cover every possible contingency here, please consider the following:

- If you're sexually active and not in a monogamous relationship (defined below), you should see a doctor or visit a public health clinic at least every six months to be tested for HIV and other sexually transmitted diseases ("STDs").
- If you or your partner is HIV-positive, discuss this together and weigh the options and various risk factors to determine the degree of risk you'll assume regarding oral, genital, and anal sex, and determine how and when you'll use barrier methods in your sexual activity.
- If your HIV or STD status is uncertain, discuss this with any new or prospective partner before you have sex for the first time, and determine how and when you'll use barrier methods in your sexual activity.
- If you or your partner has any sort of ongoing sexually transmissible condition, such as herpes or hepatitis, discuss this together and be aware of the risk factors. You should also discuss use of barrier methods in your sexual activity.
- Regardless of your HIV or STD status, an ongoing support system can help you stick to your commitments regarding safer play. I suggest that you peri-

odically review the most current literature available and establish for yourself a clear and consistent set of guidelines that you can live with. I suggest that you share your guidelines with at least one trustworthy friend, perhaps asking them to do the same with you. A mutual support network can be a helpful and very powerful tool to help you keep your play safer. Also, ongoing support groups are available through public health agencies in many parts of the United States. See Chapter Fourteen, "Resources," for suggestions. Finally, I recommend *The Complete Guide to Safer Sex*, by the Institute for Advanced Study of Human Sexuality, which contains extensive information and ideas on how to create a safer sex lifestyle; see Chapter Fourteen for this and other guides on the subject.

These are terms that may help you to communicate clearly and effectively regarding safer sex and degree-of-risk issues:

- *Monogamous* means that you and your partner have consented to be each other's sole sexual partner. You've been tested for HIV and other STDs, and you don't necessarily use protective barriers or follow safer sex guidelines.
- *Nonmonogamous* means that you have multiple sex partners with whom you may or may not have a primary relationship.
- *Nonmonogamous, fluid-bonded* means that you and your partner(s) don't avoid contact with each other's bodily fluids but practice safer sex with any other partners.
- *Polyamorous* is an umbrella term for responsible nonmonogamy, meaning that you and/or your

partner(s) engage in romantic and/or sexual involvements with persons other than just one another with mutual knowledge and consent. This can range from being a "swinger" (more focused on sexual activities than romance or long-term friendship) to "polyfidelity" (more focused on long-term, closed circle relationships usually including sex and always including deep affection or love).[5]

If you want to stop practicing safer sex with a monogamous partner, current wisdom dictates that you both be tested for HIV six months after either of you has had sex with anyone else, or after exposure to any other risk factor. If you both test negative and are mutually monogamous, then you can assume that you're negative for HIV. However, any continued risk factor, such as nonmonogamy or injection drug use, means that you can't assume that you are safe. If this is the case, continue to use a barrier method.

**Dress Rehearsal**

Try rehearsing your responses to questions you antici-

pate you may encounter when broaching the topic with your partner. Some common questions or concerns you might encounter when discussing anal sex include:

- *Why do you want to do that?*
- *I tried it once and it hurt all the next day.*
- *It just seems dirty and messy to me.*
- *Isn't our regular sex good enough already?*

NOTES

1. I have adapted this from *Asserting Yourself: A Practical Guidebook for Positive Change*, by Sharon Anthony Bower and Gordon H. Bower (Addison-Wesley, 1976).

2. There are a few exceptions. For instance, if the top feels that the scene has gone far enough, or if the top is simply getting tired or needs to refuel, those are perfectly valid reasons to stop the scene.

3. Bruce Bagemihl, in *Biological Exuberance* (St. Martin's Press, 1999), page 13: "To attract the attention and interest of a potential partner, animals often perform a series of stylized movements and behaviors prior to mating, sometimes in the form of a complex vocal or visual display. This is known as *courtship behavior*, and it usually indicates that one animal is advertising his or her presence to prospective mates or is sexually interested in another individual.... Courtship behavior is a common feature of homosexual interactions, occurring in nearly 40 percent of the mammals and birds in which same-sex activity has been observed."

4. Tristan Taormino, *The Ultimate Guide to Anal Sex for Women* (Cleis Press, 1997), page 40.

5. Thanks to Darklady (www.darklady.com) for this definition of polyamory.

# Latex and Lube

This chapter is for everyone who wants to know any-thing about using lubricant and a barrier method with anal toys and for anal intercourse. Relaxation, patience, and trust are the most important psychological tools for insertive anal sex, while lube and latex are essential physical components of safe and pleasurable anal play.

## Latex and Polyurethane

Anal sex is made more pleasurable and safe by using latex and polyurethane plastic. Even if you and your partner have made a joint decision to forego the use of a barrier in sex, there may be times when you want to use one or more types of barriers in anal sex to avoid messiness (such as transfer of fecal matter) and to make clean-up easier.

## Condoms

The first barrier method that comes to most of our minds is condom use.

Anal penetration tends to be harder on condoms than vaginal penetration because butts tend to be tighter than vaginas; thus, breakage is more likely. If you're not using enough lube, tiny abrasions (to both the recipient and the condom!) are more likely to occur as well.

The most frequent causes of condom failure are breakage and pushing the condom off the penis while thrusting so that it rolls into the receptive partner's rectum or vagina. One of the main causes of breakage is improperly rolling a condom onto an erection. If you've never used a condom before, or haven't used one in a while, try practicing by yourself first. Then you'll feel more confident and be better at it when you use condoms with your partner.

You can even take this one step further. One way to grow accustomed to the feeling of a condom on your cock is to practice masturbating while wearing one. This will also give you an idea as to how much pressure a condom can take before it breaks.

It's easy to use condoms properly if you can remember "Pinch, Place, Push":

1. *Pinch* air from the tip of the condom using your thumb and forefinger. This prevents air bubbles that cause breakage during thrusting. Some guys like to drizzle a few drops of lube in the condom tip to increase sensitivity. Drip in the lube, then pinch the tip.

2. *Place* the rolled-up condom against the end of the hard penis, making sure that the roll is on the outside, facing up. If you want a super-slick feeling against the skin of your shaft, be sure that your erection is lubed up before you put on the condom.

3. *Push* the condom gently but firmly down to the base of the penis with your free hand, unrolling it as you go. Some guys like to create a bit of "headroom" at this point by pulling up on the top inch or so of the condom—and unrolling the condom further down around the base of their shaft.

Having your partner do this for you can be a turn-on. Some folks like to roll the condom on their partner using their mouth, too. Unlubed or flavored condoms work better for this since there's no nasty taste. Otherwise, you can wipe off a prelubricated condom with a towel. Just be sure to put plenty of lube back on the outside before attempting anal penetration.

And men, while you're penetrating an anus, please check once in a while to make sure that the condom is

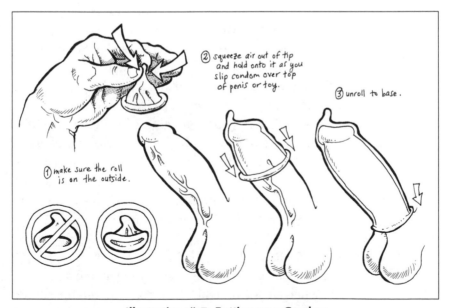

**Illustration # 7: Putting on a Condom**

still intact and on your penis, especially if you have a foreskin. Some foreskins tend to push condoms off. To be extra-protected, you can use two rubbers. Avoiding the thin variety ups your odds of protection a bit, too, although of course thickness may reduce sensitivity. Finally, make sure that the lube isn't drying out. Dryness creates condom stress and causes breakage, and it's less comfortable for the receptive partner as well. You can add more lube or simply a few drops of water to revitalize things. If you don't want to bother with handling a bedside glass, you can use a small plant mister or even a clean, damp sponge.

If the insertive partner ejaculates during intercourse, he needs to seal off the condom to avoid spills during withdrawal. (Making a "ring" with your thumb and forefinger works well.)

Condoms come in a variety of shapes, sizes, and textures. New brands and varieties are coming out all the time, and I encourage you to sample a wide array so that you may maximize your pleasure. Some recent innovations include condoms shaped for increased comfort and sensation, such as the inSpiral, which features bloated spiraling pouches that add friction and stimulation. Condomania offers a catalog that describes in stunning detail the wide, wonderful world of condoms. Good Vibrations sells a condom sampler that includes five different varieties, as well as the whole range of condoms. See Chapter Fourteen, "Resources," for contact information.

## A NOTE ON LATEX ALLERGIES

True latex allergies are rare. According to a recent study, 0.08 percent of us react to latex. Workers in certain occupations are at higher risk: hospital healthcare workers

(1.3 percent), rubber industry workers (10 percent), and dental personnel (13.7 percent).[1]

One possibility is that you're experiencing a lubricant sensitivity. Try changing your lubricant and see if the problem clears up. One gay male friend of mine was treated like a pariah at his rural county clinic over a period of months because his lube was causing his dick to break out, and the clinic misdiagnosed the problem. They thought he had some ghastly infection and gave him medication that was totally unnecessary. So lube sensitivity is often overlooked, even by medical professionals.

Many lubricants contain nonoxynol-9, a spermicide reported to kill HIV on contact. It's not uncommon for nonoxynol-9 to irritate the skin. Some people find that it makes their skin tissues go numb, too. And it's nasty stuff to get in one's mouth.

Another possibility, if you're using powdered gloves, is that you are reacting to the powder. Try using powder-free latex gloves.

Some latex alternatives are available. The condom-type alternatives are covered below. One alternative to latex gloves is nitrile gloves, which are available via the Internet or at medical supply stores. See Chapter Fourteen, "Resources," for further information.

NONLATEX CONDOMS

The Avanti is a polyurethane condom introduced in the mid-1990s. One big advantage to polyurethane as a barrier is that you can use it with *any* lubricant, even oil-based lubes that cause latex to break down rapidly. Another advantage is that it transmits heat better than latex, which can add to pleasure during intercourse. Also, the Avanti is thinner than a latex condom, which can mean greater sensitivity for the wearer. Last but not least, it provides an alternative to latex for those with latex allergies.

That said, the Avanti has several drawbacks. The most common is that, lacking the elasticity of latex, polyurethane tends to bag, which negates the increased sensitivity for some wearers. Furthermore, several studies concluded that Avanti has a higher breakage rate than latex condoms—as much as four times higher. Some users also report problems with slippage, probably due to Avanti's extra width. Finally, Avantis are considerably more expensive than latex condoms.

However, for some users, the Avanti marks a welcome change from latex or as an addition to the latex safer-sex arsenal. If you enjoy oil-based lubes, or if you have a latex allergy, I encourage you to check out this newer breed of condom.

Natural, or lambskin, condoms are also available for contraceptive purposes, but they won't prevent transmission of STDs, including HIV, in anal or vaginal intercourse.

"FEMALE" CONDOMS

The newer "female" condom, Reality, is growing in popularity, although many men, especially gay men, still don't know about it since Reality is marketed for vaginal intercourse.[2] However, it adapts quite nicely to anal intercourse. It's designed to line the vaginal walls by way of two flexible plastic rings: an inner ring that you insert into the vagina, and an outer ring that hangs outside the vaginal opening. The rings are connected by a thin, six-inch tube of polyurethane.

Since it's plastic, like Avanti, you can use oil-based as well as water-based lubricants with it. Another advantage is that you can leave it in, meaning that you can fuck awhile, stop, and then go back to fucking later without going through the process of putting on a new condom. And a lot of men prefer the sensation to the usual tight-fitting condoms.

Still, the Reality condom isn't for everyone. People who are used to condoms seem to like Reality more than do people who are used to sex without barriers. It crinkles, which some find distracting. Some guys can't get over the fact that they're basically fucking into a plastic bag, and I can't really blame them. That said, it feels better to me than a tight-fitting male condom, and I even like the look of the tube as it slides in and out with my dick. So you might slip one on and give it a test-ride.

The Reality requires a bit of patience and practice for most of us, but it can be well worth the trouble. One new user, who uses regular condoms for anal sex, reported: "It's the most sensation I've experienced on my penis during fucking since I stopped having unprotected sex in the '80s." In fact, based on anecdotal evidence, the Reality may be more satisfying for couples using it for anal than for vaginal sex. If you're a man who has trouble maintaining an erection with an ordinary condom, the Reality is certainly worth a try.[3]

Here are some tips that will help you avoid most of the snafus:

- Practice inserting Reality *before* using it for partnered anal sex for the first time. When you do use it with a partner, be sure that the condom isn't twisting. Use plenty of lube, as Reality can stick to the penis or dildo.
- The insertive partner may have to keep thrusts shallow because the condom isn't as long as the rectum, so thrusting in too deeply will stress the condom (possibly resulting in breakage) or push it inside.

- Be sure to keep the penis or dildo inside the outer ring, and check to see that the outer ring isn't being pushed up the rectum. Reality's internal ring really isn't necessary for anal sex, although it may help keep the condom from slipping out past the sphincters. Some users find the inner ring uncomfortable; furthermore, it can irritate the rectal lining and even cause light bleeding. If this is the case for you or your partner, remove the ring by reaching inside the tube and sliding it out before insertion.
- Squeeze and twist the outer ring after use to keep any seminal fluid inside the pouch, and pull it out very carefully to prevent semen from leaking out.

Typically, Reality is available in many chain drugstores, priced from five to ten times the price of a regular condom. However, many AIDS-prevention agencies, such as San Francisco's Stop AIDS Project, now distribute it free of charge, for the asking. Although it's usually sold in boxes of three (for about $9), Reality occasionally shows up in boxes of six, at a "two-for-one" price, so that's a great time to stock up.

### Finger Cots and Gloves

A latex finger cot can be used to explore the anus with a single finger. They're available from medical supply stores and some AIDS-prevention agencies. A single condom can be used to cover two or three adjacent fingers. Latex gloves are widely recommended for extended use, comfort, and the widest variety of options in anal play.

Wearing latex gloves during fingering is an effective means of protection—for both partners. Gloves can prevent transmission of bacteria and STDs to the insertive partner via tiny cuts in the hand. Likewise, gloves also protect the recipient from fingernails, jagged edges on fingers, and rough spots on hands. In addition, the hands can transmit venereal warts (HPV) from one person to another during play.

Gloves should fit snugly but not too tightly. Too-loose gloves can wrinkle, twist, and bag during play, causing discomfort for both of you. Too-tight gloves can stretch uncomfortably around the hand, restricting finger movement and increasing the likelihood of breakage.

Exam gloves are widely available at most chain drugstores, usually in boxes of 12, 50, or 100. The best deal I've found on latex exam gloves is at the warehouse stores such as Costco, where you can buy two bundled boxes of 100 gloves for about $10. That's just five cents a glove. However, as with latex condoms, latex gloves have a limited "shelf life." Plan to use any gloves that you purchase within roughly six months. As with condoms, keeping them away from heat and light will prolong their life. So store your gloves in a cool, dark place, and keep them away from oils or oil-based creams and lubes. Those zipper-lock sandwich bags make a clean, protective container for storing loose gloves.

As with condoms, not all exam gloves are created equal. Aside from size, there are other variables, including length, thickness, and texture. You may want to try several different brands to find the ones that have just the right "feel" for you. One friend who uses gloves daily in her tattooing and piercing business recommends Cranberry brand; I like them, too.

One alternative to exam gloves is surgeon's gloves. You can find a vendor by looking in the Yellow Pages under "Medical Supply." Surgeon's gloves are more expensive than exam gloves because they're sterile and manufactured to more exacting standards (the leakage rate for standard exam gloves is as high as one in four). Here's a neat trick: When you use surgeon's gloves, turn them inside out. Inflating them first makes this easier. Reversing the glove exposes the shinier inner surface, which is more comfortable to the recipient's anus and rectum. Another advantage to turning them inside out is that the gloves are longer in that direction. Turning them inside out also helps avoid the "wrinkle factor" that's especially common with exam gloves.

Vinyl gloves are generally unsatisfactory for anal play. They're not as stretchy and form-fitting as latex, so they tend to bag and crease, which creates discomfort for both recipient and giver.

## Lubricants

### Different Types and Textures

So which lube is the best lube? The one that's best for you. Individual preference is highly subjective. Fortunately, many varieties of lube are available, so you can experiment with different ones until you find your favorite. One important point is that water-*based* and water-*soluble* lubricants (such as Shaft, which is water-*soluble* but oil-*based*) are *not* the same thing! Generally, lubes can be categorized in several different groups.

WATER-BASED AND SLIPPERY
J-lube is a powdered lube that mixes with water. It was developed for veterinarians to assist in delivering newborns. J-lube is the lube of choice for many fisting aficionados, because of to its economy and texture.

It has a stringy, slimy texture that stays slippery for a very long time, but because of this, it's very odd to handle and clean up—so experiment with it a bit before using it for anal sex. Another drawback to J-lube is that you do need to mix it yourself, and you should only mix a small portion of the package at a time; otherwise, you'll end up with quarts of lube. See Chapter Fourteen, "Resources," for ordering information.

WATER-BASED AND STICKY
K-Y is the most widely available lube, but it's far from the most appealing. Somehow it never quite sheds its hospital-clinic trappings. Furthermore, as it's intended for single-use medical environments (such as the insertion of a thermometer or catheter), it's deliberately formulated to break down quickly, thus making it a poor choice for the repetitive motion of anal play.

Some folks like water-based lubes for anal sex, but for longer sessions, the gloppy lubes (such as K-Y Jelly, I-D, Wet, and ForPlay) and the sticky ones (such as Probe) tend to dry out. However, you can refresh them with a few drops of water. Generally, they make a poor choice for fisting. If you want a water-based lube for fisting, try J-lube, above. Otherwise, see the section on oil-based and liquid lubes.

OIL-BASED AND LIQUID
These include all forms of liquid oil and semisolid substances like butter and Albolene (marketed as a makeup remover) that melt easily on contact with a warm human. Oil-based lubes aren't latex-compatible but can be used quite readily for anal sex where this isn't an issue. The oil breaks down the latex, causing small fissures that can transmit HIV and other STDs. However, if

you and your partner are fluid-bonded (see Chapter Five, "Communication") or aren't concerned with small tears in a latex glove while fisting, you may want to try an oil-based lube.

Oil-based lubes encompass a wide range of substances, including any cooking oil found in the kitchen (vegetable oil, olive oil, sesame oil, and the like), baby oil, mineral oil (cheap, widely available at drugstores and warehouse stores like Costco, and marketed to relieve constipation when taken orally), massage oils, and even motor oil. (While the "grease-monkey" mechanic is a long-time staple of sexual fantasies, motor oil is smelly, extremely messy, and best reserved for external use!) Some of these oils are quite smelly, so it's a good idea to take this into account.

Baby oil often contains perfumes that can irritate some people, so if you or your partner have a fragrance sensitivity, it's best to be careful at first. Baby oil can also be too thin for successful anal sex where some viscosity is needed. However, Johnson & Johnson makes a hybrid product containing baby oil and aloe vera gel that you may wish to check out.

Albolene is an excellent lube for penile masturbation and was popularized in the gay male community during the 1980s when all-male jack-off clubs like the San Francisco Jacks and the New York Jacks were formed as group-sex outlets in response to the AIDS epidemic. Albolene also works quite well for anal penetration when latex breakdown isn't an issue.

OIL-BASED AND STICKY
The lubes in this category divide into those intended for sexual play and those that are not. Again, while oil-based lubes aren't latex-compatible, they can be useful

for activities where latex isn't involved, or where a thicker form of latex barrier (such as a glove) can be replaced periodically to avoid tears.

This group includes that old standby Vaseline. Some prefer this kind of lubricant for anal sex because it doesn't dry out (like most of the water-based lubes), plus it stays put, thus keeping the surfaces well lubricated. Cocoa butter works in a similar fashion. Then there's Crisco shortening, a long-time favorite of fisters everywhere.

This group also includes commercially prepared sexual lubricants like Elbow Grease and Shaft, which are available where sex toys are sold, often in an 8- or 16-ounce canister. These solutions usually contain various combinations and quantities of vegetable oils, glycerin, and polysorbate-80.

> **Sharing Lube**
>
> To prevent contamination of lube in open containers, such as Albolene, Elbow Grease, Shaft, or Crisco, use a clean spoon to scoop out as much as you will need into a cup or dish, and then dip into that instead of the canister. That way, you can use the same can of lube on different occasions with different partners without fear of spreading bacteria from one partner to another. This is also an important consideration for group-sex settings.

SILICONE-BASED

In my opinion, the best all-around lubes are the silicone-based ones. They work pretty effectively with everything except silicone toys—*don't* mix the two or the lube can ruin your toy! Silicone-lubes are latex-compatible yet stay slick longer than water-based lubes. At the same time, they retain some of the pleasing tactile qualities of oil-based lubes. Better still, they are hypoallergenic.

Eros, which produced the first widely marketed silicone-based lube, also makes a product called CULT

Dressing Aid for people who like to wear latex clothing. It can also be used as sex lube. Mr. S makes a similar product called Bodyglide as well as a second, Ultra Glide Gel, which is a bit less expensive than Bodyglide and is more of a general-purpose lube for anal sex. Ultra Glide Gel makes a wonderful lube for fisting! It was manufactured with this purpose in mind, and it really does the trick (so to speak). Finally, Wet, a well-known maker of water-based lube, now sells a silicone lube called Wet Platinum, a personal favorite for anal inter-course; I-D manufactures a similar product called Millennium. All these products contain dimethicone and other chemicals that can provide a barrier against latex sensitivity.

One precaution when using these lubes is that they leave a slippery residue on all surfaces. Wash thoroughly with soap and water to avoid slippage. They're also the most expensive variety of lubricant, but I think they're worth it.

HYPOALLERGENIC LUBES
Besides the silicone lubes, there's a product called Seal Skin that does what it says—it seals the skin against germs. However, it's still possible to get an *E. coli* bacte-rial infection in cuts or scratches even when wearing Seal Skin. The chief advantages to Seal Skin are that it can help assuage fear of infection *in addition* to offering latex protection, and it can prevent allergic reactions to latex for the wearer who has a latex allergy but still wants to use a latex glove for insertive anal sex.

**Be Prepared**

Making up a "sex-to-go kit" is a great idea. Keep it stocked and ready to go with you on any occasion when you might have sex outside your own bedroom. This idea is an extension of the toilet-kit bag that folks take along when they travel. Fill your "sex-to-go kit" with plenty of your favorite condoms, lubes, gloves, and small sex toys such as anal toys, cockrings, or nipple stimulators. Individual-serving packets of lube are ideal, or you can rinse out any small plastic bottle with a nonleaking cap and fill it from a larger lube container. Keep gloves in their own container, such as a zipper-lock sandwich bag. Clean-up supplies such as moist towelettes or waterless soap are useful, too. A fanny-pack makes a great container for your kit, or just use whatever you like, as long as it's easy to access at the moment you need it.

NOTES

1. www.eparent.com/resources/asktheexperts/askthedoctor_latex.htm

2. Public health professionals suggest the Reality condom for contraception because its efficacy is high. With an annual failure rate of 5%, it's somewhat less reliable than a male condom (3%) but better than the diaphragm (6%), the cervical cap (11%), or spermicide (6%). Source: Promotional literature accompanying Reality condoms.

3. For more information, visit www.femalehealth.com or call (800) 274-6601, x222.

# Tools and Toys

*I have a fairly extensive collection. It's very scary.
I keep threatening to take a picture of it and send
it to my parents.*

We live in an era of options for sexual pleasure that
would have been unimaginable even twenty years
ago. A wide variety of toys and other tools are available to you for enhancing anal pleasure. Some of
these have origins that are probably as ancient as
humankind itself, while others represent the cutting
edge of various technologies.

Many products are specifically intended for anal
sex, while some designed for vaginal penetration can be
used as is or adapted for anal pleasure. When choosing
a toy, consider what sensation you'd like: Do you want
something in your ass for a "full" feeling? Do you prefer

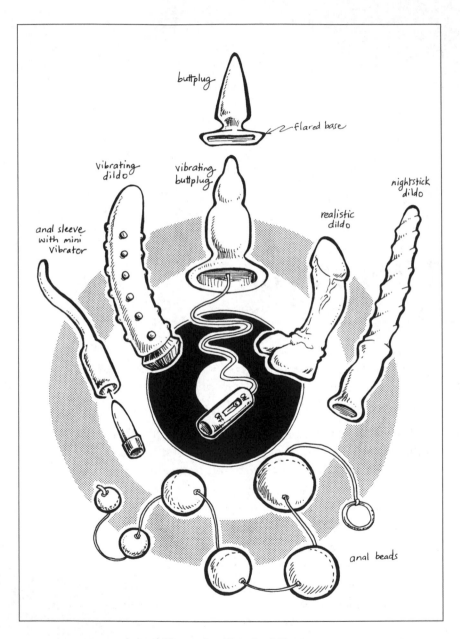

**Illustration # 8: Anal Toys**

an in-and-out rhythm similar to vaginal intercourse? Do you want your butt toy to move or vibrate?

## What Makes a Good Toy for Anal Sex?

- No rough edges or textures
- Not breakable
- Flexible
- Clean
- Flanged

Be careful of anything, be it a butt plug, dildo, or other object inserted in your butt (such as a cucumber or candle), that has no flange at its base. Essentially, a "flange" is a handle. The flange should be at least an inch wider than the rest of the toy. It gives you something you can use to pull an object out of your anus. Otherwise, you may end up making a trip to the emergency room to have it removed.

Don't ever use any object that has a sharp edge or end to it, even if you use it with the pointed side facing away. Objects to avoid include pencils, razor handles, toothpaste tubes, and frozen fish—yes, fish! See the "Curiosities and Miscellanea" section in Chapter Fourteen, "Resources," for other inappropriate items people have used for anal play!

Any object that creates a vacuum is dangerous as well. Nontapered cylinders, such as the end of a shaving cream can, fall into this category. Large blunt dildos (3 inches or more in diameter) can cause injury or get stuck if they create a vacuum. Don't let such objects into your rectum. Getting them back out is difficult to impossible. At the very least, you'll end up with a sore, scraped, and possibly bloodied hole. The rectum is quite capable of opening up suddenly and clamping shut just as suddenly. A tapered shape, on the other hand, can come out gradually.

Other considerations: Will this toy be easy to clean? Are there nooks and crevices on it where germs could hide?

The most important thing is to start small. Buy plugs and dildos that you can probably take, rather than ones you hope to be able to take. Get your money's worth out of any toy you buy.

Always think ahead in terms of your toys—plan for unforeseen uses whenever possible. For this reason, I think it's always a good idea to sheathe your insertable toys in a latex condom. You may *think* that you'll be the only one who ever uses it, but next time, someone else could be on the receiving end.

Wash your toys after use, even if you did use a barrier to keep them clean. It's not an extra precaution; it's a necessity. Many oil-based lubes (such as Crisco) will damage toys if left on them for any length of time. There's a danger of the lube providing a medium for bacterial growth. Even if you have used a barrier, some "dirty" lube will most likely be smeared around the base or elsewhere. Dawn dish detergent is popular, and an extra rinse with Betadine or Hibiclens isn't a bad idea either.

Storage is important, too. Plastic bags with a self-sealing zipper are a cheap yet effective storage method. Cloth bags with a drawstring are nice, too. Don't allow rubbery toys to come into contact with black dye, such as in cockrings, dildo harnesses, newsprint, or other toys containing black dye; the dye quickly discolors many toys.

## Butt Plugs

*You have to relax. A lot of lubrication. You may want to start off with one of the really thin butt plugs, and just maybe over half an hour, and then go from there. Slow, lubrication, and a lot of communication between you and your partner. How does the mantra go? "Communication, relaxation, and lubrication."*

Butt plugs come in a dazzling variety of shapes and sizes. The standard butt plug has an outer, flanged end that tapers down to a narrow band that's held in place by the outer sphincter, then widens again to a broad base, and usually tapers gradually to a rounded point, so that the plug is a rounded conical shape with a flat base. I have seen some that widen into other shapes, like an egg or a globe (the globe plug reminds me of a doorknob).

When you're just starting to experiment with insertion and getting comfortable with leaving something in your butt for a short while, a small, thin butt plug is probably all you need. They're inexpensive and you can always get another later if you want to graduate to something longer or wider.

Mr. S makes what I consider the Cadillac of butt plugs, an exotic-looking metal-and-rubber affair that's easy to keep inside for hours. The rubbery tube is slender and much easier on the sphincter than the traditional plug. It comes in a variety of styles: one contains vibrating metal shot (rattle, rattle!), one is attached to a cockring, and another can be hooked up to a box for electrical play. Great toys if you can afford them.

## Ways to Keep a Butt Plug Inserted

You can insert a butt plug in many different ways during solo play or with a partner. One technique that works well for solo play is to place the plug on a hard surface, such as a board, wooden chair, or floor, and to squat onto it using your hands for leverage.

Be patient. Even with experience, your outer sphincter will often resist the insertion to some extent. I recommend that you go slowly, allowing your sphincter

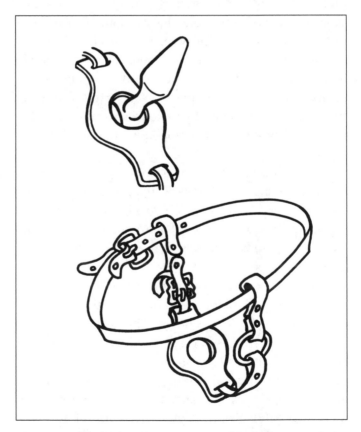

**Illustration # 9: Harness and Butt Plug**

to relax gradually, taking as many tries as you need to ease off the plug and start again.

Some people enjoy the erotic stimulation of keeping a plug inserted while going about their daily business or while out on a date (not uncommon in the gay or S/M communities). If you're keeping a butt plug in for an extended period, be sure you've thoroughly douched, because the constant stimulation from the plug can cause a peristaltic reflex, and you may need to defecate quickly and unexpectedly. Also, if you go out with a butt plug inserted, it's a good idea to take a small plastic bag (preferably the zipper-sealing style) in case you get tired or sore, or in case your sphincter starts to expel the plug. An extra pair of underwear couldn't hurt, either.

Whether you're going about your routine or have a butt plug inserted as an adjunct to a particular sexual activity (fucking, fellatio or cunnilingus, S/M play, and so on), you may want to secure the plug so that it doesn't slip or shoot out in the middle of your play. Several commercial devices are available for this purpose.

- Koala Swimwear makes a line of products with straps, including a thong harness and an underwear harness, that help keep a standard butt plug in place.[1] Thongs need to be elastic enough to snugly hold the plug, which is why the Koala devices are so good; they're designed to be functional and tight enough to hold a butt plug in place.
- Leather and fetish suppliers, such as Mr. S in San Francisco, sell a butt plug harness. The harness has a leather waistband and thong that can hold two different-sized standard butt plugs.
- Do-it-yourself solutions: A jockstrap might work for this purpose, but a thong is probably preferable because of its center strap. Some people even like

to use rope to fashion a body harness or waist harness, perhaps with knots that can hold the plug in place. Jay Wiseman's *Erotic Bondage Handbook* provides instructions for creating a rope harness.[2]

## Dildos

Dildos come in an impressive variety of shapes, sizes, and materials, ensuring that there's something to please most any butt. There are even a few folks who will make toys to your custom specifications.

### Latex and Synthetic Latex Dildos

Most mass-produced dildos are made of synthetic rubber in two colors: "flesh" and black.[3] On the plus side, they're inexpensive, they come in the widest variety of shapes and sizes, they're flexible, and they're easy to keep clean and reasonably germ-free if you cover them with a condom or sterilize them after each use. They also retain body warmth well.

One drawback to this type of dildo is that it's easy to permanently stain the flesh-colored variety. Because of this, and because the "flesh tones" are usually dreadful approximations, I prefer the black ones. The most common source of stains is ink or dye, such as newsprint, black leather—or black butt toys! Oily or greasy lube can speed the transfer of dye. So if you have flesh-colored *and* black toys, be sure to store them *separately*. You can avoid stains if you keep your toys away from inks or dyes and store them in a plastic container (such as a zip-seal bag) when not in use.

## Jelly Dildos

Jellies are made from a soft, translucent plastic called "jelly" or "jelly rubber." They come in a variety of colors, often pink. Because they're filled with little air bubbles, they are very light.

## Silicone Dildos

This type of dildo tends to be made in small batches by smaller manufacturers, and some of their creations are real works of art. They come in interesting patterns (such as marbled) and shapes (such as twisted). Strangely, silicone dildos are still not well distributed to the sex toy stores where most men shop, so many guys don't know about them. Your best bet for finding a silicone dildo is at an erotic boutique or via the boutique's website.

Silicone is different than synthetic latex in a number of important ways:

- Unlike the more common latex dildos, silicone is nonporous and cleanable. Silicone toys clean up nicely in the top rack of your dishwasher, too. You can do this with latex, but because of to their porosity they may still harbor bacteria.
- Silicone dildos tend to be firmer than latex dildos.
- Silicone is more expensive than synthetic latex, but most people who use dildos find that its qualities of matching body temperature and its general texture make it superior. Vibrating silicone dildos also transmit vibrations more strongly than equivalent jelly dildos. So silicone toys are a good example of getting what you pay for.

## Cyberskin Dildos

Cyberskin represents the state of the art in sex toy technology. It has a texture and resilience that's striking compared to conventional toys—more like that of a real penis than anything else on the market. Its variable density helps to create the more realistic effect. Of all the available substances, it warms to body temperature the most quickly. One drawback, however, is that most of these toys aren't very firm. Also, they seem to attract dirt and are difficult to clean, so you may want to cover them with a condom to make clean-up easier. However, using condoms detracts from their "real-skin" texture. If you're using a toy made of cyberskin only for your own pleasure, simply washing it with water and antibacterial soap may suffice. Allow it to dry thoroughly before storing or reusing—almost all microorganisms that cause problems in the human body require moisture to live, so drying your toys is a very important precaution.

# Vibrators

One of the lesser-known benefits of vibrators is that they help relax the anal muscles. Vibrators come in plug-in and battery-operated types.

Battery-operated vibrators have the advantage of portability, but they tend to be less durable than the plug-ins. Because of their low cost, though, there's a huge array of novel battery vibes, such as the Hello Kitty vibrator available from Toys in Babeland and other stores. I have only seen some types of vibrators in a battery-operated style, such as vibrating butt plugs. (However, the high-end electrical boxes designed for sex play usually have optional butt plug attachments that you can purchase separately.)

The Hitachi Magic Wand, a high-end vibrator, is the most popular vibrator at San Francisco's Good Vibrations. It's a plug-in style with a rounded head that you can use externally—on the anus, perineum, testicles, a partner's clit, or anywhere you please. Some people even use it on the neck and feet! Of course, you can also use a vibrator to get an extra buzz out of an already inserted dildo or butt plug.

While you can't use a large wand-style vibrator internally, an attachment is available for the Hitachi Magic Wand, called the Wonder Wand, that fits over its head and provides a four-inch dildo for vaginal or anal penetration. There's also a curved extension for wand vibrators, called the "G-Spotter," that will deliver vibrations to the prostate.

You can experiment with the position of the vibrator, too. Try shifting it around to vary the sensation. Use it on your scrotum or perineum in conjunction with anal or penile stimulation.

## Specialty Toys

### Double-Ended Dildos

The safest double-ended dildos have a bulb in the middle that keeps one orifice from contacting the other.

Partners can penetrate each other simultaneously with a double-ended dildo. Also, a woman can use a double-ended dildo in the butt and in the vagina at the same time. However, she should avoid placing a dildo in the vagina once it has been in the anus, as this spreads intestinal bacteria to the vagina, which can lead to infections.

### Inflatable Dildos

Good Vibrations, Mr. S, and most of the specialty stores listed in Chapter Fourteen, "Resources," carry this unique expandable device, which can add an extra dimension to your butt play. Inflatable dildos are made of rubber and contain a bulb and a hose with a stop-valve to maintain a specific level of inflation. Some aficionados assert that these toys are useful for increasing one's capacity to take larger objects, such as a hand, into the rectal cavity. As with any anal activity that pushes the limits, however, use prudence during any experimentation, and don't do too much too quickly in the heat of passion. Inflatable dildos have been known to tear and collapse due to over-inflation.

### Anal Beads

Just what they sound like, anal beads are a series of "beads," or balls attached to a cord. They're gradually inserted into the anus—many people like to yank them out during orgasm. For safer sex reasons, anal beads of this type are a single-user toy and shouldn't be shared. Make sure the "beads" are smooth—no rough plastic seams—and the cord is firmly attached.

A type of thin-shafted dildo called a Prober is also available that has a series of small, molded balls along its shaft, which can function similarly to a string of anal beads. These are made by Falcon and available on their website (www.falconstudios.com/falcon/shoppers.htm) and other sex toy websites and shops.

### Chrome Eggs and Butt Plugs

Toys such as chrome eggs and butt plugs thermally conduct very well. Some users like the contact of the cold chrome as it slips inside them. Most users, though, will want to touch them to their skin to warm them before insertion into an orifice. Chrome absorbs and re-radiates energy (heat or cold).

Since chrome eggs lack a flange, they should only be used by experienced players who know their limits. Be sure that you can sterilize them thoroughly before sharing them with others. Retailers who sell these toys should be able to advise you on how to do this safely.

Don't release steel or chrome toys—including cock-rings—into the toilet because they will crack the porcelain! Even if you intend to grab the toy as it falls, it will be very slippery and can easily slip through your fingers.

## Electrical Toys

> *It's a real good fuck. When I get what I call my "zapper box" going, it feels like I'm plugged into the fucking universe, it makes my butt so happy!*

With an electrified anal plug or probe, you can always get a rhythmic fuck when a lover is too tired, unavailable, or nonexistent. The advantage over a regular dildo is that you can adjust the speed, rhythm, and intensity to your precise liking and keep your hands free for stimulating other erotic zones. An electrified fuck can be hard, fast, and repetitious; or soft, slow, and gentle; or anywhere in between, in any combination. A drawback to these toys is that they're expensive. Another is that the wires limit your mobility during play.

The star of the "electro-stim" system is the metal control box. Various attachments can be plugged into the control box to stimulate the rectum, anus, penis, scrotum, nipples, clitoris, urethra, or vagina. The ever-increasing number of electrified toys designed for safe anal play attests to the growing popularity of penetrative anal sex. See Chapter Fourteen, "Resources," for vendors who can provide you with additional information on these specialized systems.

Electroplay is a specialized form of sex with a breadth beyond the scope of this book. If you're interested in exploring further, I recommend the book *Juice* by "Uncle Abdul"; see Chapter Fourteen, "Resources."

Electroplay systems can be used for pleasure or pain play, depending on the attachment, how it's used, and the intensity at which it's used. For additional information on the latter, see Chapter Eleven, "Extreme Sex."

## Harnesses

*At this time of my life, I actually prefer strap-ons to dicks. One thing is the disease factor in this day and age. Condoms do break.*

Strap-on play isn't just for women anymore.[4] Think about it, guys: With a strap-on, you can temporarily have a dick of any size or shape you like. A strap-on can add variety to your sex play; even many men who fuck their partners regularly with dildos never think of harnessing them. And last but not least, you can give Mr. Happy some down time while continuing to satisfy your partner.

*I find women with strap-ons extremely hot. Especially the ones who like to let their hair grow in various places. It just rocks my world.*

Harnesses let women *and* men wear a dildo or vibrator over their pubic bone or thigh to penetrate their partner, while leaving their hands free. Some harnesses come with a built-in dildo or vibrator, while others have rings, straps, or other ways to hold a separate dildo.

Thong and jockstrap style harnesses are widely available on the market; men should probably go for the jockstrap models. There are also jockstrap style models that hold the dildo higher on the belly, which fit larger men and women quite nicely.

The "Thigh One On" straps onto the thigh rather than the hips. Two partners can each wear one and slide between each others' legs to allow penetration; this can work better for simultaneous penetration than trying to use a double-ended dildo. You can try strapping the Thigh One On above the knee, too—the flexible position of the jointed knee acts as a fulcrum, allowing for rotation in and out, plus finer motor control than you can get by using the hips in conjunction with the thigh.

Standard harnesses have moderate-sized rings, usually up to 1.5 inches in diameter. It's important to make sure that the harness you select will hold the toy you want. Some harnesses can accommodate wider toys, while others are made to hold a variety of ring sizes. If the harness ring is attached with snaps rather than rivets, you can change the ring to a larger size. You can also use rubber or neoprene rings that will stretch to hold a larger toy. Most of the sex toy stores listed in the Chapter Fourteen, "Resources," sell larger steel rings as well as rubber or neoprene rings. You could also try a hardware store to see if there's anything ring-shaped there (large key rings, napkin rings, curtain rings, large rubber grommets, and the like) that will fit the bill.

A final resort is to have a harness custom made. Most leather shops serving the fetish community should be able to help you. Finally, Mr. S has a self-harness that comes with two different attachments for different size plugs. They also make a harness that's adaptable to virtually any dildo; ask them about the D352 strap-on belt.

## Cleaning Toys

You should clean and disinfect any butt toy before inserting it—or use a condom on toys during play as a less labor-intensive alternative. (By the way, this is a good use for expired condoms—you can use two layers to be extra-safe.) However, I like to do all three steps and recommend that you do, too. For the first step, clean your toys with hot water and a liquid pump antibacterial soap such as Dial. Next, to disinfect them, cover and soak toys for 10 to 20 minutes in a solution of 1 part bleach to 9 parts water, or full-strength Betadine (povidine iodine), hydrogen peroxide, Simple Green, or Hibiclens. Iodine works best if you let it dry on the toy's surface. Isopropyl alcohol is good at removing skin oils and the material trapped in them, but it is not going to disinfect your toys. You can also use a commercial sex toy cleaner, although they're often pricey.

Third, silicone toys can be run through the dishwasher (which uses the hottest possible water, depending on your water heater's setting) or boiled up to three minutes to disinfect them. Boiling doesn't disinfect rubber and synthetic rubber toys, since they're porous. However, some people like to preheat their toys in a large pot so that using them is more comfortable. Don't stick hot toys in your butt, though. Keep toys no more than a few degrees above body temperature.

If you try this trick, just be careful to keep an eye on things—I'll always remember the time that a friend's large and cherished rubber dildo melted down into the bottom of the pot! (It made a great conversation piece, though.)

If you want to share your rubber and synthetic rubber toys with others, either put condoms on them or switch to silicone dildos. For more delicate synthetics, such as cyberskin (made from thermal gel), stick to warm water and antibacterial soap, and replace them every so often, as they're impossible to keep perfectly clean.

Never submerge the battery or motor part of a vibrator in liquid. These are notoriously fragile toys, and you don't want to shorten their already brief life expectancy. Don't submerge electric vibrators at all. Using condoms and cleaning with antibacterial soap and hot water afterward is a good compromise. (Scrubbing for two minutes is recommended.) You can use a latex glove to cover the noninsertive larger vibrators (such as the Hitachi Magic Wand) during use.

While we're on the subject of cleaning, you can clean up leather harnesses with a damp rag (reconditioning the leather if it gets dried out). Just toss nylon-web harnesses in with the rest of your laundry.

## Shopping

You can buy dildos and other sex toys, as well as condoms, lubricants, and other sex supplies, via the Internet—but hands-on shopping is definitely preferable for any type of toy that you're buying for the first time. The look and feel and heft of a toy should be important to you before you lay down your cash. The usual outlets are:

- Adult book stores, also known as "adult video stores" or "porn arcades." While some of these stores are worthwhile places to shop, at most of them the toy selection is small, overpriced, and often of questionable quality. The lighting, design, and display of merchandise seldom provide a comfortable, relaxed shopping experience. The staff is occasionally knowledgeable, but usually their chief function seems to be to keep the furtive from walking out without paying for their goods. Alas, this is still how much of America shops for its sex toys.

• Leather stores, which have been a fixture in the urban gay male community for years. These stores are attracting more and more shoppers of all orientations as kink busts out of the closet. The staff ranges from knowledgeable to "decorative," but the environment is generally more comfortable and sex-positive than in the adult video stores. The anal toy selection is usually decent but varies from store to store. Generally, they're a good place to buy male-oriented sex aids such as cock toys and anal beads, as well as more exotic toys such as urethral sounds and butt plug harnesses. Most stores have one or more craftspersons who can make alterations to leather harnesses, clothing, and toys, or can offer custom work to help you fulfill your fantasies.

• Erotic boutiques, also known as "sex toy stores." Many cities have at least one nowadays, such as Good Vibrations in San Francisco and Berkeley, Grand Opening! in Boston, Toys in Babeland in Seattle and New York City, and many others. In contrast to the traditional adult book store, typically these stores are woman-owned and operated, the design and lighting of the store are intended to enhance your shopping experience, and the staff is knowledgeable, helpful, and trained to put you at ease.

If you don't live near one of these stores, however, fret not. Along with the traditional mail-order catalog, the Internet has evolved into a state-of-the art way to purchase toys and other supplies for sex. There are many advantages to shopping via catalog or on the Internet: anonymity, confidentiality, and the certainty that your purchase will arrive in a discreet wrapper. One big point in favor of the Internet is that it offers a way to view the latest offerings from the online emporiums (sex toy stores, leather stores, and so on) that might not appear in the same store's printed catalog for a year or more.

In her seminal book, *Good Vibrations: The New Complete Guide to Vibrators,* Joani Blank suggests that you "check the return policy of any company you're ordering from. A reliable company should accept returns of defective vibrators for at least thirty days.... [I]f you want to find out more about the company, ask how they choose toys, or how long the company has been around." To avoid unscrupulous cyber-shops on the Internet, she recommends that you "look for a site that provides some sex information along with its products. This is one indication that a company is genuinely interested in people, not just money. Look for a toll-free number and mailing address on the web site."[5]

### Cruising for Toys

If you're not sure what toys you'd like and your local porn shop doesn't stock any but the most common rubber toys, you can take a virtual shopping trip: shop till you drop! Check out Mr. S (www.mr-s-leather.com), Mercury Mail Order (www.mercurymailorder.com), or any of the other sex toy shops featured in Chapter Fourteen, "Resources."

## NOTES

1. www.koalaswim.com or (800) 238-2941.

2. Jay Wiseman, *Jay Wiseman's Erotic Bondage Handbook* (Greenery Press, 2000), pages 232–38.

3. A British company, Creative Mouldings, manufactures an extensive line of high-quality black latex toys that I like—molded dildos and plugs made from a hot-melt, vinyl-based rubber compound. Several U.S. retailers, such as Mr. S in San Francisco, carry its inventory. Check it out at http://dildos.co.uk.

4. For further information on strap-on play, see *The Ultimate Guide to Strap-On Sex*, by Karlyn Lotney (Cleis Press, 2000), and *The Strap-On Book*, by A. H. Dion, (Greenery Press, 1999).

5. Joani Blank and Ann Whidden, *Good Vibrations: The New Complete Guide to Vibrators* (Down There Press, 2000).

# Tongue in Cheek: Analingus

Also known as rimming or anal/oral sex, analingus involves stimulating the anal region with the mouth and tongue. Often this is combined with genital or other forms of stimulation, since rimming is in itself a fairly mild form of stimulation. Still, when stimulated, the nerve-rich skin around the anus is a source of pleasure for many of us. Few people can orgasm by analingus alone, making it mostly an adjunct to other forms of sex that many find enjoyable. Some people enjoy analingus as a prelude to anal intercourse as well.

One positive thing about rimming is that you don't really have to worry about the possibility of hurting your partner, as with anal penetration. But the anal taboo certainly extends to rimming (we don't generally say "Kiss my ass!" as a come-on!), and besides, there are health risks to consider before leaping tongue-first into the fray.

## Doin' It

If you're trying out rimming a partner for the first time, work up to it gradually and see how they react. You can start with cunnilingus or fellatio and work your way down. Many people find rimming a turn-off, at least initially, so don't assume that you can just dive in full-speed-ahead. In fact, if you're having comfortable

---

### Especially for the Novice

If your partner strongly desires analingus but you don't feel comfortable giving it, you can exercise your right to refuse. If you're worried about weird smells and tastes, you can ask your partner to wash before starting. You can even do it yourself if you share the shower. That's a romantic way to segue into it.

You can try drizzling a bit of honey or syrup between their buttocks, or try a flavored lube, available from a sex toy store, and see if you like that. Remember that oil-based lubes will destroy condoms, so if your plans include anal penetration, stick to the water-based flavored lubes.

Your partner may want analingus but be shy about mentioning it to you. Notice their nonverbal cues during sex—do they arch their back toward you, nudge your head lower, or raise their butt when you're giving them oral sex?

If you've never done this before, share that with your partner. They will probably tell you what they like—and if they don't volunteer this information, ask. If you're on the receiving end with a novice, be patient, and don't make them do anything that makes them feel awkward or inadequate. A little encouragement usually goes a long way.

discussions about sex, you can say that you'd like to try licking or chewing their butt and see how they react. Some people think it's "naughty," so if you get that reaction, you'll have to gauge whether that's a good "naughty" or a bad one.

In fact, you can incorporate the naughtiness factor into your play. If verbal sex turns you on, you can talk dirty to your partner about what you're doing to them down there. Tell them what a naughty girl or boy they are for liking this. Have them ask or even beg you for more.

It's usually a lot easier to access the anal region if one of you uses your hands to spread the cheeks. What you do then is up to you, and there are a lot of variations and countless combinations of them all. Some people prefer a light flicking motion. You can vary the speed to see what turns them on the most. Some folks like to be probed as deeply as possible, with the tongue held rigid and pushed firmly inside. Or you can just push gently at the anus with your tongue. Making a smacking sound with your lips as you press them against the anus ("puckering against the pucker") can create pleasurable sensations, too. Some people even get turned on by the noise this makes. You can also try humming or moaning as you are licking them—the vibrations will transmit to the receiver, who might get even more turned-on!

Another stimulating method is to widen the tongue and apply pressure over the entire outside area. You can nibble lightly around the edge of the pucker. Or you can try sucking or biting on the hole, but proceed cautiously at first, as not everyone likes these more intense kinds of stimulation. Everyone's turn-on is unique, so pay close attention to any physical or verbal cues you get.

## Get Comfy

Rimming is often a prelude to penetration. Many people who like to be on top during anal intercourse get very turned on by starting out this way. Whether rimming is a prelude to other forms of penetration or the main event, the person rimming will want to be as comfortable as possible. Otherwise, you'll tire out after a couple of minutes. A comfortable position for the neck is essential. Usually, this involves the recipient's butt being at the same height as, or slightly above, the rimmer's mouth. Here are some positions you can try:

### Recipient on knees, kneeling in front and facing away.

This is an easy position to hold on a mattress, and it works even better if the recipient can crouch low in front, so that their weight is resting on their shoulders rather than the elbows. This allows easier access for the rimmer.

### Recipient on back, buttocks elevated.

If they're limber, they can probably rock back and hold their ankles close to the head for up to a couple of minutes. Other possibilities include suspending the ankles by way of straps hung from the ceiling, or by using a sling: a suspended piece of leather or network of ropes or straps. (It's a little like a hammock for sex—in fact, most hammocks could be adapted quite readily for this activity.)

### Recipient on side, buttocks extended.

This is the rimming equivalent of "spooning," where partners lie on their sides with the front partner's backside nestled up against the back partner's front—like spoons nestled in a drawer. For rimming in this position, the person rimming will probably want a pillow under the neck if they wish to hold this position for more than a minute or two.

### Recipient seated, rimmer facing up.

Folks who enjoy analingus have devised various contraptions involving a hollowed-out seat that allows the rimmer to position themselves beneath the butt. One such device, the Joy Rider, is a professionally marketed, durable product that some analingus aficionados enjoy. Essentially, it's a high-quality toilet seat mounted on springs and a pipework frame that's high enough for someone to scoot under and service the person seated. Mr. S and some of the other suppliers listed in Chapter Fourteen, "Resources," can provide you with further information.

## Health and Risk-Reduction Considerations

It's unlikely, though theoretically possible, to transmit HIV via rimming. Complicating factors could include the presence of fecal matter or anal fissures and ulcers around the rimmee's anus, or cold sores, cuts, or bleeding gums in the rimmer's mouth.

However, the real health risk involved in rimming is the transmission of parasites and hepatitis (see Chapter Thirteen, "Anal Health," for a detailed discussion of each). While there's no way to make rimming totally safe, aside from use of a barrier (which I'll discuss in a moment), you can reduce the risk of transmission somewhat by observing the following precautions:

- The main risk is contamination with feces. Rimming a clean butt is less risky than rimming an unwashed one, especially after a bowel movement. Some people like to douche before being rimmed, although this isn't necessary. Douching will reduce but not eliminate the bacterial population in the rectum. Washing the butt with antibacterial soap and water before rimming is sufficient. You can use a moist washcloth or a medicated pad such as Tucks, or a baby wipe if it's not soaked in alcohol (alcohol can sting and cause anal itching). Don't use anything that will be unpleasant to taste, and avoid any paper that falls apart, such as toilet paper—the flakes won't enhance your erotic experience! Wipe gently but firmly; you don't want to create irritations or tiny cuts that could become infected. It's probably best to avoid perfumes—again, avoid alcohol around the anus. And if you're planning to have anal intercourse using latex condoms, don't use aromatic oils or oil-based lubricants, which weaken latex.

- Shaving or trimming the hair around the anus helps keep it cleaner and reduces the risk of chafing the lips. (If there's stubble, however, it can cause abrasion more quickly.)
- Deep probing with the tongue held rigid is probably riskier than just lightly flicking the skin around the pucker.
- Another option is to navigate around the anal sphincter instead. The fleshy cheeks of the butt, the perineum, and the scrotum are also filled with nerve endings that are sensitive to tonguing, sucking, and biting. Many of us love having attention devoted to our perineum—in men, pressure also stimulates the prostate and scrotum indirectly—yet our perineal pleasure potential is often overlooked in the focus on the genitals and anus. Sucking or biting the

perineum is worth trying, too. So you may even draw a bigger reaction from your partner from tonguing the perineum than the sphincter. Pay attention and notice which activity draws the most intense reactions.

## Using a Barrier

Let's face it—almost everyone into rimming would rather tongue a clean, fleshy hole than a piece of latex. Using a barrier diminishes the taste, smell, and feel of the anal region for the rimmer. The person being rimmed usually experiences reduced sensation, too. Nonetheless, a barrier is a safer choice when you're concerned about your partner's health status (or your own) and still want to indulge your penchant for rimming.

Good Vibrations gives a big "thumbs-up" to Glyde brand dental dams. Dental dams are 4-inch squares of latex originally designed for use in dentistry. Glyde and other manufacturers have redesigned them for sex—making them larger and thinner, and even adding various flavors.

In a pinch, you can also use a condom that's been slit up the side with the tip snipped off. There's also household plastic wrap—use the regular, nonmicrowavable kind. The wrap made for microwaves is porous, which defeats the purpose of using a barrier.

Be careful when using barriers that you use the same side consistently! Some folks mark one side with a permanent marker to make it easier to tell which is which. If there's any doubt, switch to a new barrier.

**Kiss, Kiss**

Experiment with a partner, using different forms of analingus: kissing, light flicking, deep probing, licking with a swiping motion on one side, then the other, and so forth through many delightful variations. You can also try light spanking or spreading their cheeks apart with your palms before delving in. Try each kind of contact for at least ten or fifteen seconds before switching. See which motions provoke the most pleasurable reactions, judging by their moaning, breathing, talk, and body language. You can ask for feedback afterward.

# Penetration

*You can get a blow job from anybody, but when it comes to anal intercourse, the closeness is intense. It's just a different level of intimacy.*

*I'll feel a really good fuck in my ass for hours afterward. Just real tingly, it'll be puckering for four to six hours.*

## For the Insertive Partner

Fucking ass can be just as much fun for the receiver as for the giver, but most people need to learn how to be penetrated comfortably. There are many ways to make anal penetration easy and enjoyable, but perhaps the most important of all is to experiment with yourself before you try penetration with a partner for the first time.

In your preparation for penetrative play, wash your hands, remove any rings, and trim and file your finger-nails. Rough spots, such as hangnails or the skin that sometimes collects and hardens at the corners of the nails, need to be trimmed and filed away. Ideally, you shouldn't be able to feel the edge of the nail with the pad of your thumb or index finger if you've done a good job. Calluses can be softened somewhat with skin lotion.

While latex or nitrile gloves can cover a multitude of sins, it's best not to rely on them to ensure a smooth entry. The sensitive anal opening can still detect a sharp edge through a glove. Furthermore, as with douching, trimming and filing one's nails can be useful as a medi-tative process to prepare oneself mentally as well as physically for penetrative play. In fact, some people enjoy doing this preparation in front of or in conjunction with their partner, because it heightens the anticipation.

### It Starts with a Finger...

*Make sure you do a lot of anal massage. The Body Electric tapes are so great. Or any kind of training on opening up the whole area slowly and lovingly so that you're really ready before penetration. Start with a finger, and lots of lube, and work up to bigger objects. Take your time.*

Each of us is unique in terms of how we like to be touched. The anal region is no different in this regard. Furthermore, each of us may like different kinds of touching and stimulation at different times. Most people find it pleasurable if their foreplay includes lots of

touching of the entire body—touching that's not necessarily sexual or genitally focused, but that encourages
relaxation and builds trust.

> *People don't give enough emphasis to exterior*
> *butthole massage. Play with it. There are a ton of*
> *really good nerve endings there, and there's a*
> *delicious point of noninsertion. Just massage and*
> *enjoy it.*

Some of us prefer smooth, outward strokes in a
gradual stretching of the tissue around the sphincter.
Others enjoy circular strokes, with an occasional finger
slipping just inside the outer sphincter. Still others prefer a repetitive in-and-out motion to stimulate the
outer sphincter muscles. You may discover that your
partner enjoys all three at varying points during anal
play. It's vital that the receptive partner communicate
his or her preferences, discomforts, and turn-ons, particularly in the "getting-to-know-you" phase of the sexual relationship. Often a few clear words make all the
difference between a delightful time and an awkward
experience.

The person doing the touching can ask for feedback, too, particularly if their partner isn't communicating much. Ask your partner what kind of motion feels
best. Is it friction or fullness that gets them the hottest?
How about the position, angle, and speed? Does your
partner enjoy genital stimulation during butt play? Self-
stimulation or from you? How about nipple play? Do
they want lubricant on or around their hole? How
much? Perhaps a gentle neck massage or shoulder rub
with your free hand? Do they like it when you lie on top
of them? Don't be afraid to shift, but be sensitive, and
don't make changes too abruptly. Slight changes can

make a huge difference in the receiving partner's experience. Both partners need to take their time, stay relaxed and present, and communicate.

And, by all means, switch roles if you wish! Or you can try simultaneous touching and stimulation. There's no reason one person should get all the attention—unless, of course, that's what you've planned beforehand.

Work up to anal touching by touching other parts of the body first and then gradually incorporating playing with the anus. You can stimulate your partner's genitals as you begin to touch the outside of the anus. Gentle but steady pressure (without penetration) and then stroking away from the center of the pucker with the pad of the thumb or forefinger can be a pleasant way to begin. Another method is to slowly circle the pucker with the pad of the finger, using light pressure. Also, some people enjoy analingus (see Chapter Eight, "Tongue in Cheek") as a way to open up their partner's hole as a prelude to penetration.

You may want to do this for a while before attempting any penetration. If your partner is new to anal sex, you might even keep the anal stimulation secondary to genital stimulation the first few times you experiment with it, and forego penetration until you both agree that you want it. Even without penetration, there's a difference in sensation between pushing the area around the anal opening and pushing right in the center, so experiment with that and pay attention to your partner's reactions. If his or her pucker begins "winking" at you, regard it as a good sign! Avoid any sudden or jerky movement. Any friction will probably communicate as unpleasant stretching, so be sure to use enough lube for anything more intense than light touching.

There are many approaches to penetrating the sphincter with a finger, and the best way to find out what works is to talk to your partner. Sex educator Robert Lawrence[1] recommends the simple "flick-up" technique, used by doctors for putting a finger into a butthole during rectal exams: Begin by rocking the pad of your finger against the anal opening as you bear down. It doesn't matter whether you flick from above or below the hole; just don't bend the finger as you flick it into the hole. And, of course, you're using plenty of lube for this, right?

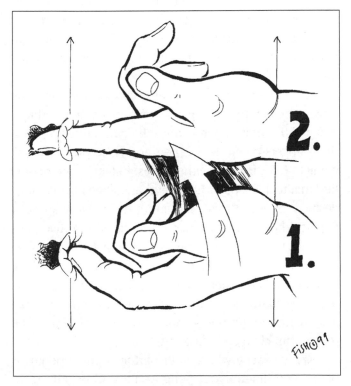

**Illustration # 10. "Flick-up" Technique**

Work up to the point where most or all of the finger is sliding comfortably in and out of the butt. Many people enjoy the sensation of a finger pressing forward, toward the front of the body, along the inside wall. Experiment gently with this. For many men, this stimulates the prostate; many women enjoy this stimulation as well, since this wall is the other side of the thin vaginal wall and contains a great many nerve endings. In fact, if you use the other hand to finger inside her vagina, you can feel the finger pressing against the other side of the wall.

Just don't use the same hand to play with both the vagina and the rectum. If you must, then make absolutely sure you can keep track of which finger was inside her butt and which was inside her vagina. The rectum contains bacteria that can cause infection when introduced into the vagina.

Once the receptive partner is comfortable with one finger, you can try adding a second finger, and perhaps, if that's still comfortable, a third. If your partner can take three fingers comfortably, then he or she probably isn't going to have trouble with a penis. In fact, some people find that taking a penis is easier than taking fingers, since fleshy penises are softer and more malleable than bony fingers. The main difference is that if the insertive partner is on top, then there will be considerably more pressure from fucking, since much more weight will be behind the movement. This is one reason why some receptive partners prefer to start by squatting over the insertive partner's penis. Another is that this puts the receptor in charge, feeling safe.

Know exactly where your partner's anal opening *is* before you slide in your penis or a toy. One good technique is to place a fingertip into your partner's relaxed sphincter and use it as a guide so that you know where to slide in. You can also have your partner help guide you in, since they know what hurts and what doesn't.

*Avoid rushing. Even with somebody who's very eager and quick, rushing is a mistake because once you rush too fast, they really shut down and it takes a long time to get past that.*

One technique for insertion that works well for many folks is to use a slight pumping motion with the hips while pushing very gently at the anal opening without actually penetrating it. After a minute or so, you can start to add a tiny bit more pressure each time. You should take several minutes to achieve full penetration with this method. This gives the receptive partner a lot of time to relax—your partner can use the relaxation tips in the next section.

Remember that you can incorporate other types of stimulation during all of this. You can play with or massage your partner's genitals, nipples, back muscles, and so forth. You can use your free hand to massage, slap, or otherwise play with your partner's butt cheeks while you're playing with their hole or penetrating them with a penis, fingers, or toys. One "sweet spot" that a lot of folks don't know about is the cleft running vertically between the visible end of the tailbone down to the anal opening. Pressing or rubbing this part of the body can be delightful for the receptive partner.

*When I'm doing the inserting, I'm aware of giving somebody pleasure that's very personal. For me, it's similar to the pleasure I get when I give somebody a good massage—the feeling of rubbing flesh that I'm stimulating in a nice way. And butt-*

*holes are like that, but more concentrated. And they're muscular, so you get instant feedback on what's going on.*

*There's usually a fairly tight feeling when you're in someone's ass. Vaginas aren't typically that tight. Yes, I love a vagina, too, but an ass is just more familiar, and it feels a little better, too, because it's more snug.*

## For the Receptive Partner

*When something hits my prostate, I get an overall tingling sensation that I find really hot. Kind of over my whole body, but really centered in the anal area.*

*I didn't used to think that anal sex was clean or sexy, but now I realize that most reasonable men would enema or douche before they do that, so that's not a problem anyway whatsoever. Works for girls, too!*

## The Anal Essentials: Communication, Relaxation, Lubrication, Trust

It's important to take things slowly. In fact, many folks need to practice self-stimulation before attempting partnered anal sex. Take your time and experiment with different positions and angles. Don't be afraid to stop your partner as often as necessary to make adjustments. You'll feel more comfortable and experience more pleasure—and ultimately, so will your partner.

Don't be afraid to guide your partner's penis or toy into you so that you can adjust the angle and rate of penetration, especially when exploring anal penetration with a partner for the first time. It gets easier with familiarity. Talking about the sensations as you try different approaches helps your partner learn your body.

Don't stimulate your own penis until after you have comfortably accommodated your partner's penis or toy. Arousal causes the anal sphincter to tighten up and can make penetration more difficult.

> *There are guys who are really lousy at fucking, and I've found a few, mostly when I was younger. You need to find guys who know what they're doing.*

One common misconception is that penetration is "supposed to" hurt at first until it gets comfortable. Pain is your body's way of telling you when something isn't right. There's no reason why anal sex should hurt the receptive partner. You wouldn't start a physical workout without warming up and stretching your muscles; likewise, you may experience less discomfort if you ease into getting fucked. Yet guys, especially, are raised to believe that they should "tough it out" and not complain when they feel pain. This is macho nonsense. Honesty and communication are essential ingredients in negotiating successful anal intercourse (not to mention life in general!).

## Three Relaxation Techniques

- One way to allow penetration is to make a slight pushing motion, as though you're having a bowel movement. Much of the bowel movement action is really just a relaxing of the anal sphincters (peristalsis), whereas the internal intestinal pressure is what actually pushes out the waste.

- Another technique is to ask your partner to insert very slowly as you take deep breaths. Keep your shoulders relaxed as you do this. Once he's inside you, just have him rest there while you relax and adapt to the sensation. Again, allow the process to take as long as it requires. You're more likely to have comfortable, pain-free intercourse if you start out easy.
- Some receptive partners, particularly more experienced ones, like to take the penis all at once and then just relax around it. Squatting over and sitting on the insertive partner's penis is a favored position for this. The trick is to use deep breathing and to insert as the receptive partner exhales.

### Motion and Position

Some people find that an in-and-out motion is uncomfortable to accommodate, particularly if the insertive partner's penis is unusually straight or stiff, or longer than five or six inches. One solution is to have the insertive partner use a circular rather than a thrusting motion for penetration. You can also ask him to use shallower strokes until you feel comfortable taking more depth. Be sure to use plenty of lubricant, on both the inserter's penis and in the recipient's rectum. Don't be afraid to push the lube past the sphincters using your fingers. Keep a towel handy to wipe off any excess.

There are many different positions you can try to achieve greater comfort; squatting, for instance, allows a greater degree of control for the receptive partner than doggie-style or the traditional missionary position. Most people squat facing the insertive partner, but you can experiment with squatting while facing away as well.

Some people find that lying on their side, facing away from the insertive partner (also known as "spooning"), is the most comfortable position, and since this is a common sleeping position, it allows the body to relax fairly completely.

Everyone is different, though. Once I was having anal sex with my male partner, who wanted to penetrate me from on top, in the missionary position. This is a position that's often troublesome for me as the receiver. However, I found that by resting one leg over his shoulder, and letting the other rest on the bed, it felt fantastic! And I've never seen that variant described in any book or website on anal sex. So it's very important to experiment and learn what works for *you*. See "Positions to Try" below for more ideas.

Don't allow yourself to be penetrated longer or faster than feels comfortable. It's important to pace yourself! Some people find it essential to take frequent breaks. Don't feel self-conscious or worried about your partner's disappointment. Stop as often as you need to in order to enjoy the experience of being penetrated. Sometimes you may feel as though you need to squat on the toilet, or switch to a less intense type of penetration (such as stimulating the opening with your own fingers), or just need to stop to slow your heartbeat. Knowing that you can stop when you need to is essential to developing trust—and the right to say "STOP" goes for insertive as well as receptive partners!

As you and your partner develop communication and trust regarding anal intercourse, you'll develop your own intuitive rhythm as a couple. As you gain experience with receiving anal penetration, and in particular as you learn to relax, most likely you'll find yourself enjoying the sensations for longer and longer periods of time.

## For Both Partners

### The Joy of Simulated Penetration

Some find the mere motion of a body *simulating* anal penetration to be a tremendous turn-on. Like the anus, the perineal ridge that runs between the genital region and the buttocks is filled with sensitive nerve endings. A partner can insert his penis between the receptive partner's legs and hump away. Add a bit of lube if you wish. With reasonable prudence, you don't even need condoms. This can be as orgasmic and as intimate as actual penetration for both partners.

To keep play safe, you need to be aware of the following:

- In the pleasure of the moment, the insertive partner may say, "Well, I'm not going to fuck you, but I'm going to just stick the tip in"—this still constitutes unprotected intercourse. Any STD that can be transmitted via deeper fucking can also be transmitted via insertion of the head of the penis into the anus.

- The insertive partner is at risk as well as the receptive partner. In rubbing around someone's perineal region without wearing a condom, you may get a speck of shit in your urethra and get a nasty urinary tract infection (UTI). "I was on this transcontinental flight, and I had a painful, demanding urge to pee every fifteen minutes," recalls one unfortunate recipient of a UTI. If this occurs, see your doctor immediately.

- If no condom is used, both partners should wash off afterward.

## Be Aware of Risk Factors

Fucking without a condom, with or without ejaculation into the rectum, is still considered dangerous. In one study, the risk factor for HIV dropped from hundreds of thousands to one down to hundreds to one when a condom wasn't used.[2] Tiny tears in the rectum or penis can serve as portals for the transfer of HIV or other STDs. Pre-come can carry the same viral load of HIV as semen (ejaculate). The difference would be in the amount of infectious material, since most men ejaculate one to two tablespoons of semen while considerably less pre-come.

Some people are being less cautious overall, now that there's medicine to slow the progression of HIV. For instance, in group sex settings, a careless person may stick a finger up someone's butt, and then put the same finger into someone else without cleaning it first. This is an easy way to transmit intestinal parasites as well as anal warts and other microbial meanies. So be careful in group settings, such as parties and sex clubs, that no fingers or other body parts stray where they don't belong. You and your sex partners should wash up before playing whenever possible—preferably showering with antibacterial soap. Don't forget to rub the soap under the fingernails as well as over the genitals and anus.

The same is true of toys: Sharing undisinfected toys is a quick route to infection. You risk spreading any bugs that are in your partner's ass into yours. Even if they're not STD bugs, plenty of others can wreak havoc. Clean any toys thoroughly before sharing; you'll find instructions in Chapter Seven, "Tools and Toys." And see Chapter Thirteen, "Anal Health," for further information about HIV and other STDs.

**Positions to Try**

Initially, at least, the receptive partner should be in charge of the scene, since they're the most likely to experience pain or discomfort. The only exception I can think of is where both partners have agreed to be "consensually nonconsensual," in a domination or sadism context. (See Chapter Eleven, "Extreme Sex" for further information.) However, in all cases, communication is the key to finding and refining the positions that work best between two partners. Height, rectal anatomy, mood, current physical state, time constraints, and many other factors all play a part in what works—and what doesn't succeed one time may be just fantastic the next. Keep an open mind.

## MISSIONARY POSITION

The receptive partner lies on their back, legs spread or knees pulled up. The receiver can rest their ankles on inserter's shoulders, or the inserter can hold up the receiver's calves or shins. If a sling with straps or stirrups is available, the receiver's ankles can rest there instead. Place a pillow or two under the receiver's butt (covered with a towel, perhaps) for optimal angle and maximum comfort, easing the strain on the lower back over prolonged intercourse.

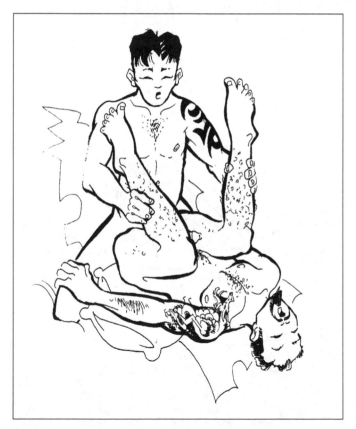

**Illustration # 11. Missionary Position**

## DOGGIE STYLE

Receiver rests on elbows and knees, and inserter enters from behind. Some support, such as pillows or a bolster, can be used under receiver's chest or belly—perhaps under the elbows, too—so that they can relax more. Receiver's chest and head can be on the mattress with arms splayed out, so that the back is arched. Doggie style can be difficult for beginning receivers since it offers a penis or toy the deepest access of all the positions. But don't be afraid to experiment with this position, which offers a lot of flexibility.

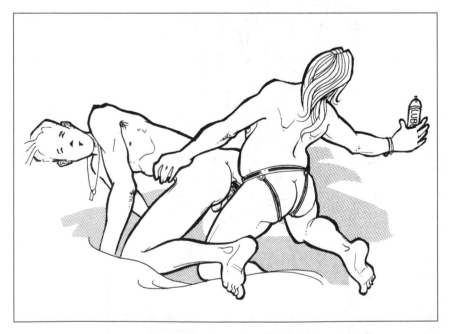

**Illustration # 12. Doggie Style**

## SPOONS

So named because partners are positioned to fit together like spoons in a drawer. Receiver lies on their side, knees bent, back to inserter, who duplicates receiver's position. Receivers may find this position easier than others. Because the degree of penetration is a bit less, it prevents the inserter from going too fast, and since it brings the inserter closer than with other positions, it makes it easier to read the receiver's reactions. Also, for recipient men, it tends not to hit the prostate directly.

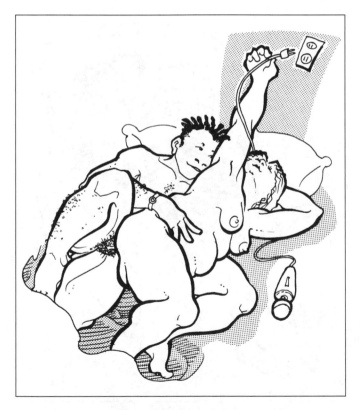

**Illustration # 13. Spoons**

## SCISSORS

Partners lie on their sides facing each other. Legs are in a scissors position. Receiver extends upper leg into whatever position is comfortable and affords access to the anus—in front of them, or held up with free hand, or held up by inserter. Upper leg can also be drawn up toward the chest or bent straight upward. More complicated than most positions.

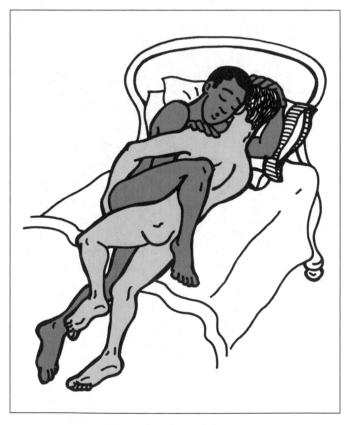

**Illustration # 14. Scissors**

## SQUAT

Receiver on top, squatting on top, either on knees or on feet, is often the easiest position for receivers since it offers the greatest amount of control. Breathing deeply helps you to relax; the inserter may nudge inward on the exhalations, once the receiver is comfortable with the sensation. Generally, if you are comfortable and relaxed at the time of intercourse, you will not feel queasy and sore later.

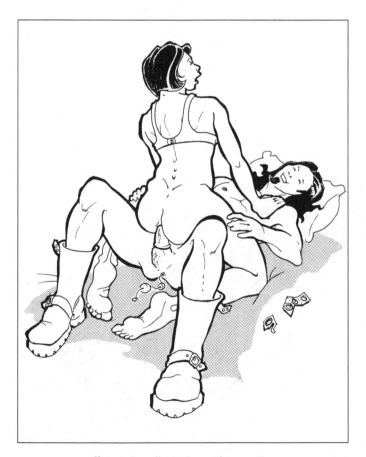

**Illustration # 15. Squatting on Top**

LAID-BACK

Both partners lie on their backs, facing each other, in a kind of flattened-out variation of the squat, with the receiver's anus over the inserter's penis. Both partners can be supported by pillows as necessary for comfort.

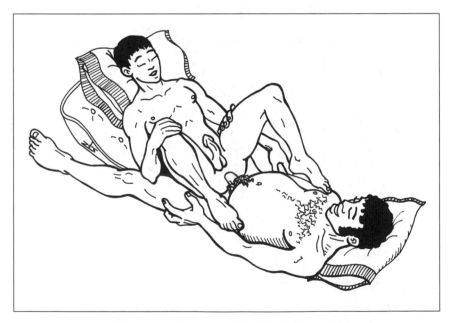

**Illustration # 16. Laid-back**

## STANDING

This is an erect variant of doggie-style. Receiver stands in front of and facing away from inserter. Receiver will probably bend over a bit to make access easier. Receiver braces against a wall, dresser, doorway, or bed. Useful in the shower and in public lavatories!

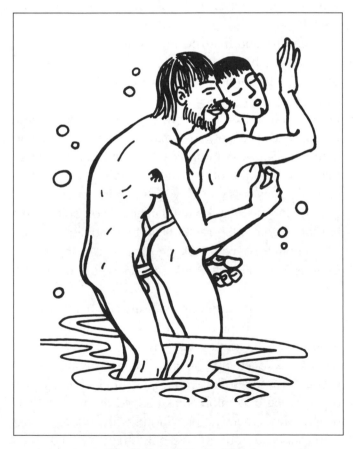

**Illustration # 17. Standing**

## Discomfort and Relaxation Techniques

Some people report feeling queasy or sore after being anally penetrated. Often, physical discomfort comes from not feeling completely relaxed at the time of intercourse. Most people find that they prefer certain positions when being anally penetrated. It's important that the penis, dildo, or other object enters and moves at a comfortable angle; otherwise, it runs into the rectal wall, which can cause discomfort, even tearing and bleeding.

Bear in mind that the rectum isn't a straight tube, and that its shape and elasticity vary from person to person. So be careful with insertion until you learn the location of the first rectal curve in your partner. If you notice a pain deep inside when you are being pene-trated, that's probably the source. You can help elimi-nate the pain by communicating with your partner so that they're aware of its location and can avoid irrita-tion. Also, any toys you play with should not be so rigid as to hit the curve at a painful angle. If you hold excess tension in your pubo-rectal sling, that can also increase the amount of pain. Doing Kegels can help; see Chapter Two, "How It Works, and How to Work It," for details.

Farting happens during anal sex, and it's best to be matter-of-fact about this. It's nearly inevitable for the receiver to fart in some situations—basically, any time air has been pushed up the butt when inserting toys or cocks. This can also happen during an enema. If you're experiencing discomfort from trapped air, try breathing deeply while crouching on all fours with your ass higher than your head. You can push outward with your anus on the exhalations. You can also try lying on your left side.

Some discomfort can occur simply because a certain amount of air gets pumped into the anal cavity during penetration. Of course, other factors that have nothing to do with sexual activity can affect the digestive tract as well. See "Avoiding and Dealing with Gas" in Chapter Four, "Hygiene and Diet," for further suggestions on how to deal with this.

## After Sex

It's important to be careful when removing a condom so that you don't drip, slosh, or spill its contents into the anal canal. When withdrawing your penis, hold the open end of your condom around the base of your dick by making a "ring" with your thumb and index finger and withdrawing slowly. If using the Reality condom, squeeze and twist the outer ring to keep any fluid inside the pouch.

Men and women alike should urinate after having sex. Peeing flushes out the urethra, which helps avoid irritations to it, such as from lube, and reduces the incidence of STDs.

NOTES

1. Private conversation, spring 2000.

2. "Sexual Transmission in the Era of New Treatments," Liz Highleyman, *BETA* (Bulletin of Experimental Treatments for AIDS), summer 1999, 12:3, 12–21. See in particular the chart on page 15.

# Fisting

*The handball experience is based on trust. A bottom must be able to trust the top with his very life. This is not something that everyone can do. A top shares a great degree of intimacy with his bottom. After all, the bottom is, in a way, revealing his very soul to him. Finding a person with whom you can share this intimacy and trust is very rewarding. Handball allows you to drop all facades and just be you. In handball the bullshit of life disappears.*
—R. A. FOURNIER, "THE INTELLIGENT MAN'S GUIDE TO HANDBALL (THE SEXUAL SPORT)" [1]

Anal fisting, also known as handballing, is the gradual insertion of an entire hand, perhaps even the arm, into the rectum.

One popular misconception is that "fisting" is literally what it sounds like: making a fist and jamming it up someone's ass. It's actually more like starting with a single finger and adding one finger at a time until you end up with your hand in the shape of a cone, and gently pushing into the receptive partner's anus and rectum.

Like other forms of anal sex, fisting doesn't have to hurt at all—most folks agree that if there's pain, then your ass isn't ready. Nor is your mind, since mental preparation is vital. I have played with beginner bottoms for whom the mental barrier was the greater one. In all honesty, however, some people do work through some degree of discomfort to "stay with the scene" and go on to be successfully penetrated with a hand. Still, it's vital to respect your body's limits and know when to stop. This is truer of fisting than any other form of anal sex, and this is why everything we've covered regarding communication applies doubly when it comes to anal fisting.

Fisting releases a flood of endorphins—proteins with strong analgesic (painkilling) qualities—in the fisting recipient. The emotional highs (and lows) that come about with the sudden generation of so many endorphins can be overwhelming for the fisting recipient. Crying, laughing…fisting seems to be an unusually potent emotional act for many people. This may be akin to the effect some chiropractors have discovered, whereby placing a few ounces of pressure on a specific point at the base of the spine can cause immense emotional relief.

Someone who accepts a hand into their butt is expressing a profound degree of trust in the partner. When fisting is done with sufficient preparation, care, and precautions for safety, it can be a pleasurable, intimate, even spiritual experience for both partners. For some, it's the most intense erotic experience they ever have. Fisters often describe the experience using quasimystical terms like "extreme intimacy," "erotic meditation," "merging with my partner," "becoming one with the universe." So fisting is all about feeling, in both senses of the word—intense emotions as well as intense sensations.

## Myths about Fisting Dangers Persist

It bears repeating: Fisting is *intense*—emotionally as well as physically. Many people practice other types of anal sex for years before they even attempt it. Along with communication, everything I've said up to this point regarding safety, hygiene, preparation, and penetration is doubly true when it comes to fisting.

Few sex acts are more widely and deeply misunderstood. The 1980 Al Pacino movie *Cruising* probably did tremendous damage to the image of fisting in the public consciousness by misrepresenting it as an act of violence. Furthermore, fisting achieved a reputation during the early days of the AIDS epidemic as a highly dangerous activity, a misconception that persists to this day. However, most of the fisters who contracted AIDS during the 1980s were also practicing other high-risk behaviors and didn't understand how to take precautions to minimize the health risks. These risks come from three areas: body trauma, infection by HIV and other microorganisms, and drug abuse.

### Not Just for Gay Men

As with other forms of anal sex, fisting is widely believed to be exclusively a gay men's sexual activity. While gay and bisexual men did popularize the practice in the late 1960s and 1970s, it has been practiced by people of all orientations for thousands of years.

As with any form of sexual activity, if you can think of doing it, chances are good that someone's getting off on it right now, and that people have been doing it for ages. Perhaps the only relatively "new" forms of sex arrived with the advent of new technologies—electricity, silicone, computers, and whatever's next.

Breaking a taboo often carries a great attraction. The lure of the forbidden is powerful and, paradoxically, many of the most banned and profane acts are turned into quasisacred elements, especially in outcast cultures, such as the widespread adoption of fisting as a sexual activity by many gay men in the late 1960s and 1970s. Fisting has, in fact, been a part of the human sexual repertoire since time immemorial—there are descriptions of the act in ancient Hindu texts—but in our culture, it took an outcast culture of gay men to popularize an act that was almost unknown, or at best considered profane, and transform it into a ritual that many now consider sacred.

## Prepare Yourself

### Find a Quiet Setting

Having a peaceful place to play uninterrupted is important. If you play music, choose music that's soothing and relaxing, preferably instrumental, set at a level that is low enough for the players to hear one another easily. Music should probably not have a beat that's too insistent or dominant. There's lots of room for your imagination here. Appropriate ambient music, "New

Age" music, discs of nature sounds, solo instruments, "world" music, classical music, and mellow jazz are some possibilities. High-energy dance music is probably not a great idea, as you want to set your own rhythms.

Similarly, lighting should be low and indirect, but not so dim that you can't easily see your partner's face or anything that you may be using with your scene, like lube or toys. Some people find that warm lighting colors, such as red or amber, are conducive to creating the desired mood.

### For the Receptive Partner

A calm preparatory mood begins with your cleansing routine. Rinse internally to clean out fecal matter, which can cause abrasions and infection. Most experienced fisting bottoms wouldn't dream of presenting themselves uncleansed to a top. It can take several cycles of filling and emptying to get clean, but don't overdo it. Allow extra time to relax and unload additional retained water. Preparation via proper diet and other factors can make a big difference here; see Chapter Four, "Hygiene and Diet."

### For the Insertive Partner

Fingernails can cause a serious perforation. If you're putting your fingers into a butt, your fingernails should be short and filed down so that you can't feel the edges when you scrape them against your opposing palm. Pay particular attention to the corners, where it's easy for sharp edges to hide. Rings should be removed and stored in a safe place. All of this preparation is a good idea whether or not you use gloves, and besides it will put you in the mood! It's always acceptable for the bottom to inspect the top's hands, and doing so may help the bottom feel more at ease.

### For Both Partners

Some people like to do yoga stretching or other exercises designed to limber up their bodies and help them focus. You may find that meditation, focused breathing, or some form of ritual helps you to "draw a veil" between the mundane world and the ecstatic, erotic world you're about to enter. It doesn't matter whether you do this alone or with a partner, although sharing the experience can be yet another way to build intimacy.

### TAKE YOUR TIME

A very important factor to success is to have a relatively unlimited amount of time. Fisting is rarely a "quickie" activity, even with the most experienced partners. Plan to allow at least two hours for play.

### DON'T BE GOAL-CENTRIC

Having the proper mind-set is essential for fisting. For all comers, it's important not to be goal-oriented. In this case, the journey *is* the destination. How far you get isn't the point. Some fisters won't even dignify the question "How far are you in?" with an answer. Getting a hand all the way into your butt doesn't confer on you any mystical wisdom, worldly knowledge, or sacred intimacy unavailable from other parts of the experience. In fact, you're more likely to achieve some of these things by focusing on the overall person, not just on the activity.

Partners may feel compelled to go further than they really want to, just because they're trying to impress the partner or exceed their own previously set limits. How far you get on a given occasion depends on any number of factors over which you may or may not have control, such as experience level, current level of stress in your life, fatigue level, general health, degree of comfort with your partner, size of the fister's hand, and so on.

HAVE CLEAR COMMUNICATION WITH YOUR PARTNER
It's essential to be up-front and clear about your level of experience. Mutual honesty and trust are fundamental to a successful fisting experience.

Establishing eye contact and "ear contact" are crucial to gaining the kind of deep connection described above. While gay male erotica involving a blindfolded or bound fistee in a sling can make for hot one-handed fiction, in real-ity most people require the moment-to-moment feed-back that comes from a constant connection. You should be able to make eye contact and hear the other person's voice and even breathing. Those inserting shouldn't be afraid to ask *lots* of questions, particularly in the initial stages. Eye contact is vital to draw the other person into your mind-space. Take your time and do whatever it takes for the two of you to be in sync.

> **To Increase Your Receptivity**
> Practice with fingers and dildos. Some people practice for years with fingers and dildos just to get fucked, let alone fisted. You can also use a vibrator to help relax the anal region. Butt plugs work for some folks, too. With either dildos or plugs, you can increase the size and width as you become more comfortable.

## Tools and Tips

### Slings

A sling is a suspended, reclining support made of leather, canvas, or nylon that allows the receptive partner to lie on their back with the head above the waist, giving the insertive partner easy access to the genital and anal regions, and providing the receptive partner with enough support to completely relax. A sling can be a single-piece construction (like a hammock) or many perpendicular straps riveted together in a web. Slings are usually hung from hooks or O-rings bolted into posts, overhead beams, or the ceiling, but some self-supporting units come ready to hang from their own framework.[2]

This specialized piece of equipment is available from leather stores, erotic boutiques, and the like. As with other sex toys and furniture, you can even order slings via the Internet nowadays (see Chapter Fourteen, "Resources," for a listing of vendors), although, as with a bed, it's important to test a sling by lying in it to see if it will be a comfortable shape and size for you. Some fisting aficionados find that adding a pillow under the head makes for a more comfortable experience, especially for prolonged scenes. It's also important to have straps to support each ankle, and straps for the hands aren't a bad idea, either, since they can provide leverage if the receptive partner needs to shift around.

A sling isn't necessary for fisting; in fact, many fistees prefer to be positioned on a bed, "doggy-style" on their knees, which keeps the rectum and colon in the straightest possible position and often permits the greatest depth.

### Lubricant

There should be no friction when fisting. Use liberal amounts of lubricant to ease entry and keep things running. The favorite for fisting is still vegetable shortening such as Crisco. (I'm told, however, that Safeway's house brand has less odor than Crisco.) J-lube is probably the next most popular fisting lube. Commercial preparations such as Elbow Grease and Shaft also have their fans. You can purchase these in plastic cans of various sizes at many sex-toy and leather stores, or through the mail and over the Internet. Some folks like cocoa butter or mineral oil. In general, water-based lubes are inadequate. You can also use some silicone-based lubes, such as Mr. S Ultra Glide Gel. Avoid any substance containing perfumes or other additives that can irritate the sensitive anal lining. For this reason, products containing nonoxynol-9 are *not* recommended.

What's the best lubricant for fisting? Simple: the one that works best for you and your partner. While Crisco and J-lube seem to be the most common, opinions vary widely among fisters. Most find the greasy kinds much better than water-based lubes for any prolonged action. Silicone-based lubes seem to work fairly well, too, although you'll want to use more than you would for other activities like intercourse or jacking off. Whatever you use, it's important to have lots of it on hand (so to speak), and if you're using water-based lube, you can remedy its tendency to dry out by sprinkling or spraying the area with water. Some folks even keep a small plant mister bedside for just this purpose.

See Chapter Six, "Latex and Lube," for a complete description of the various types of lubricants.

### Gloves

Using comfortably snug latex (not vinyl) gloves is a great idea. Gloves cover a lot of rough spots on hands, particularly hardened skin around nails. In practice, however, some fisters don't use gloves. At major fisting clubs, gloves are provided and often required. Some receivers find the rubbing sensation irritating (although sometimes this occurs in conjunction with water-based lube, which, as noted above, isn't ideal for fisting), and inserters usually experience a decrease in sensitivity. In general, both parties report a reduction in the degree of intimacy experienced. So discuss up front whether or not you'll wear latex gloves.

If you're sensitive to latex and want to use gloves, you'll be glad to know there are some outstanding nonlatex gloves available. See Chapter Fourteen, "Resources," for information on how to obtain these.

If you're using latex gloves with an oil-based lube, such as Crisco, the oil can eventually break down the latex. It's a good idea to change the gloves every fifteen minutes or so.

Gloves need to fit. They should be neither uncomfortably tight and constricting, restricting movement, nor too loose, as this causes bagging and wrinkles in the glove that can feel uncomfortable to the receptive partner. Plus, the top will have less sense of touch.

IF YOU'RE NOT USING GLOVES
- Nails need to be clean, trimmed, and filed. This is a good idea even with gloves.
- The top shouldn't have any fresh cuts in his or her hands. Note that the top could have microscopic openings in the skin around the base of each fingernail that may permit entry of bacteria, viruses, and the like.
- When the rectum or colon has been stretched by fisting, finger fucking, or penetration with a penis or dildo, there are often microscopic tears. That is why fucking someone without a condom, after fisting, is a bad idea. This is a really large window of opportunity for the transmission of STDs. Of course, one

alternative is to fuck first, fist later; another is simply not to fist and fuck on the same day.

## Play

Every handballer develops their own style of play over time. The most important thing is to do what feels safe and natural, and to pay exquisitely close attention to the receiver's responses.

Begin by opening the hole following the directions in the previous chapter on penetration. When you reach the point where you're working three or more fingers inside the hole, you can progress to using the whole hand. Form a cone by aligning the fingers, either straight or gently curved, and tucking the thumb under them. You can use two basic techniques at this point: twisting and straight pressure. Some respond better to one than the other, while others require a combination of the two.

### Twisting

Slowly work the hand against the resistance of the hole, making eighth to quarter turns. As you push into the hole, increasing pressure, twist the hand slightly. Usually the hole slowly opens up and allows more of the hand inside.

### Straight pressure

Hold the hand steady and apply ever-increasing pressure to the hole. Your partner will probably tell you to ease up at some point. Relax the pressure on the hole, but don't unnecessarily pull the hand back. When your partner's ready, gently start increasing the pressure again.

Gentleness and patience are key at this stage in the process. Pay attention to the signals the bottom is giving you, as well as to the signals the bottom's hole is sending you. Follow the natural curvature of the anal passage. You can wiggle your fingers slowly to open the butt wider, gently massaging the anal walls. Broaden the fingers slowly as the bottom relaxes, and avoid sudden movements.

When you reach a point where the sphincter is about to slide over your knuckles, a push from this point will take your hand inside. After the anus crests the ridge of your knuckles, the path of least resistance is for your hand to slide all the way in. Often it feels like the anal muscles are literally sucking you in. For your partner, there's a great release of pressure and an ecstatic rush as the hand makes this passage. It's a mind-blowing experience, especially for newer bottoms.

Once your hand is inside, hold it still. Take a few breaths while you regard your partner. If they seem to be in another world, pause for a few seconds and keep your hand as still as possible before moving it again. At this point, the slightest movement of your hand is magnified immensely.

Encourage your partner to breathe deeply. This may take anywhere from a few seconds to a couple of minutes. Then proceed slowly, allowing your partner to direct the action. Sometimes you may reach a point (perhaps a curve in the rectal wall) where it just seems logical to curve the fingers around the thumb into a fist.

The passage into the anal canal is really controlled by two sphincters, an inner and outer anal sphincter (as discussed in detail in Chapter Two, "How It Works, and How to Work It"). Until the bulk of your hand makes it through both of them, your partner won't feel the release and will experience some discomfort. It may feel to you as though your hand has made it into the hole, but if the narrow part of the wrist hasn't passed the inner anal sphincter, your partner will feel as if you've stopped with the wide part of your hand still stretching the hole. That's not comfortable at all. One test is to go in and then pull back just slightly. If you're all the way in, you'll feel the inner sphincter wrapped around your wrist at the very base of your hand. Asking your partner is always a winning technique as well.

Remember to help your partner adjust and relax by encouraging them to breath deeply and evenly.

Keep an eye on the amount of lube. You should keep adding lube to your hand, your wrist, and your partner's butt as you insert deeper.

If the receiver is new to handballing, the feeling of sliding over a hand and resting on the inserter's wrist will be very new and highly intense. As the inserter, it's part of your responsibility to take your time, keep your movements minimal, and talk the receiver through the sensations. If you have any doubt about how quickly to proceed, *slow down.* You can always ask the receiver whether they want you to change the speed. In time, the intensity of entry diminishes, but it's important to remember that the new receiver isn't used to having the anus and rectum stretched to such extremes.

Accordingly, the novice receiver may want the inserter to remove the hand immediately upon insertion to the wrist. However, removing the hand can be as intense for the receiver as inserting it. In fact, if your partner is new to being fisted, you may not get back in if you pull out right away. Thus it's important not to withdraw too quickly. Deep breathing accompanied by slow, deliberate withdrawal is the safest, most comfortable choice. If the inserter breathes in time with the receiver, this can relax and restore confidence on the part of the receiver. Eye contact is good, too.

Presuming that the receiver wants to continue, there are a few basic techniques that the inserter can use to stimulate the ass. These include the *twist,* the *shimmy,* the *piston*, and the *bellows*. The twist involves rotating the fist in a circular motion so that the anus rubs against the wrist and the rectum rubs against the changing bulk of the fist. The shimmy is carried out by rapidly vibrating the fist; the fist isn't moved, just vibrated—you can tap the forearm of the inserted hand with the loosely clenched fist of the other hand, and the resulting vibrations will transmit to your partner's ass. The piston involves moving the fist in and out of the rectum in a fucking motion; advanced players often enjoy having the fist come completely out and then back in. The bellows involves opening and closing the fist slightly to increase the feeling of bulk.[3]

## Some Tips and Tricks

- The receiver needs to choose a comfortable position. Many prefer a sling, although some would rather be on their hands and knees.
- The inserter can use a vibrator on the receiver to help relax the anal muscles.
- The inserter can use his smaller hand. Right-handed people usually have smaller left hands.
- While in a sling, the receiver can crunch forward into a U shape as if she or he is doing sit-ups. Do this slowly, as the inserter's hand can get sucked up rather quickly. This works especially well when the receiver's on the verge of taking the hand all the way inside.

- For the moderately advanced, another technique is to bear down as if trying to take a shit, clenching the lower abdomen. Don't strain hard, but gently bear down. This is particularly useful for people trying to gain depth beyond the rectum.
- The receiver needs to relax and trust the inserter. While it's hard to stay relaxed when being stretched to your limits, this is important. If you're are in a sling, you can relax your entire body by making sure your shoulders are relaxed. Let your shoulders fall toward the floor. And as always, you can practice deep breathing regardless of your position or type of penetration.
- Always have a roll of paper towels nearby to facilitate clean-up. Disposable underpads, or "chucks," are great for fisting, too. These are plastic-coated on one side and absorbent on the other. Ask your drugstore or a medical supplier about them.
- Another option is to purchase a rubberized play sheet from one of the vendors listed in Chapter Fourteen, "Resources." A much less expensive alternative is a piece of easy-to-clean, medium weight, smooth black Naugahyde or vinyl upholstery fabric, available at many fabric stores for under $20.

## Masturbating While Fisting

Some bottoms like to stimulate themselves while being fisted, whereas others can develop the ability to have an orgasm, or even ejaculate, without even touching their genitals. Some tops like to masturbate the bottom with one hand while fisting with the other hand. Masturbation can play a widely varying role in handballing. Some points to consider:

- The top should ask up front, before starting, if jerking off the bottom (whether male or female) is OK, and then start slowly.
- Some male bottoms prefer that their dicks be kept dry and free of lube. Ask before you grease it up.
- Jacking off (or "jilling" off) could be a dangerous distraction if the receiver becomes genitally centered, thus interrupting the feedback mechanism to the butthole.
- A top who's masturbating could find his or her balance affected, plus the jerking off motion also transmits motion to the other hand. Rapid jerking-off motions aren't appropriate when you have a hand inside your partner's body.
- Be aware that the top's concentration may be somewhat diluted.
- Stimulation of the penis or clit can cause the butthole to tighten up, impeding progress.

## Urinating During Fisting

The bladder is located directly above the rectum. Handballing stimulates this organ and may create a need to urinate. A few receivers may find themselves urinating involuntarily. The best way to prevent this is to urinate before beginning handball play. Otherwise, keep an empty pitcher or basin nearby, plus a supply of paper towels. Of course, if both partners think that water sports play is hot, you may choose to incorporate this into your scene.

## Varying Levels of Experience

Let's examine the four possible scenarios involving experience level between two partners. While it's difficult to draw a line between "experienced" and "not experienced," I'll use those terms here to distinguish between someone who's well versed in fisting and someone who's a relative newcomer.

Whether you've had an entire hand in your butt or have had your entire hand in someone else's butt can also make a difference in terms of how much sensitivity you've developed in the practice of fisting. Ideally, both participants should learn this activity from those with experience.

More than any other butt-sex activity, fisting tends to be extremely mutual, with "switching" (each partner on the receiving end at some point during the scene) being fairly common. Please bear this in mind below where I use the terms "top" and "bottom" for the sake of brevity.

### Neither Top Nor Bottom Experienced

Don't expect to do it all or go all the way on the first date. Start with just a finger. Have no expectations. The bottom should have played a lot with fingers and perhaps toys before attempting to be fisted.

As a novice bottom may fear injury, so may a novice top fear injuring the bottom. If you're both inexperienced, get someone experienced to coach you if at all possible. Experienced teachers go a long way toward dispelling insecurity and fear. It really is best if at least one of the partners has received a fist previously, but if this isn't the case, *proceed with caution.* If you approach handball with the gentleness, patience, care, and respect—and even reverence—that it demands, and if you're prepared to spend time getting there slowly, you won't hurt one another. If you can get yourself to any sort of fisting demonstration or seminar, it will help you tremendously. Check with your local leather or S/M club. If they don't already sponsor demos, perhaps they can be persuaded to organize one.

If you're a novice, your partner needs to know that. Handballing is one sexual activity you can't fake your way through. Control over the scene should always lie with the bottom. A good top (or top-in-training) will stop when the bottom tells him or her to. Don't worry about looking stupid or inadequate. Neither of you should be afraid to talk or ask questions.

If you've agreed to use safewords in your play, it's important for the top to honor that. Regardless, a loud, clear "STOP" means "stop what you're doing right now." Tops, don't let your ego or your desire for a deep connection—no matter how strong, and no matter how close you are to being wrist-deep in that butt—override your better judgment. This is doubly true if you're on any kind of perception-altering drug. In fact, fisting tops have no business using such substances; to do so is to court disaster.

That said, there are some fisting sadists who do enjoy pushing the limits of a masochist's anal pain threshold. I have known some couples who agree in advance to be "consensually nonconsensual" in this way. To my knowledge, the bottoms haven't been seriously injured. This is a rare case, however, and it occurs between people who have a lot of history together. If there's any doubt in either partner's mind about how far to push things, then it's paramount to honor that doubt and take it easy.

I have also been in rare situations with a partner who asked me to back off when my hand was so close to being inside that I knew it would be easier to complete the entry than to back off. In other words, it was better to allow the sphincter to narrow and clamp around my wrist than to back off, which would have stretched the sphincter more by pulling it back over the widening part of my hand. The way I dealt with this was to hold still and have us take some deep breaths together. Fortunately, this did the trick. It had a little bit to do with luck and timing, and more than a little bit to do with our high level of shared experience.

## Top Experienced, Bottom Not Experienced

In this case, the bottom needs to be honest about his limits and not try too hard to please or impress the top. The top needs to proceed with great care and delibera-tion. Neither one should be goal-oriented. Tops will be more successful if they get feedback, back off when nec-essary, and provide opportunities for rest. If the top is used to more experienced players, he or she shouldn't project those expectations onto a novice.

The top should orient the bottom beforehand as to any advice or tips that he or she wishes to impart. Both should discuss their feelings, particularly any fears or concerns, *before* the scene begins. This can save a lot of difficulty later on.

## Bottom Experienced, Top Not Experienced

Here the bottom needs to give the top a *lot* of guidance. For example, talk about technique and types of motion. What feels good in your butt and what doesn't? How fast should the top go? What's the appropriate rate of insertion? How much can he or she rotate the hand? Is it OK for him or her to wiggle the fingers? How much lube should be used? What's the appropriate angle of the hand or arm?

The top needs to be at one with the bottom in terms of being able to pick up subtle clues, such as body movement, breathing, a quick look of panic on the face, a jerking of the extremities because something is suddenly painful. "OUCH!" is very effective communication! And, again, "stop" means stop *now*.

### Top and Bottom Both Experienced

Go for it! However, just because you're experienced, don't throw caution to the wind. Proceed with the usual attention to common sense when you're entering new territory or playing with a new partner. Experience can produce complacency, and this isn't good when you're trying new things. Also, don't assume that just because your partner is experienced, his or her activities and preferences complement yours. Fisting encompasses a wide variety of techniques and is definitely not a one-style-fits-all activity! Discussing your likes and dislikes beforehand is still important. Feedback during the scene remains important as well. Be sure to check in with your partner, take breaks for drinking fluids (especially if you're using drugs), and take responsibility for your own overall physical comfort. Because fisting can be such an all-consuming activity, it's important to pay attention to energy level.

### And Regardless of the Context...

*It's a team effort, but the bottom should provide the guidance, and the top should be receptive to this guidance and act on it.*

## Withdrawal and Beyond

After orgasm, or when either partner indicates the session is finished, allow the hand to slide *slowly* out of the anal cavity. The bottom may try and push the top's hand out very quickly. This is often an involuntary response, like shitting. The top should resist this. Hold the hand steady until the bottom can release the hand in a more controlled manner. The inserter should never pull, nor should the bottom push; that is one way to tear rectal tissue and cause injury. Instead, the receiver should breathe slowly and deeply, remaining relaxed. The ass knows how to expel what's in it; just let the process take its own time.

You'll want towels, either paper or cloth, close at hand for clean-up, along with a trash receptacle. Commonly, the top will clean the bottom. It's a good idea to have water or juice nearby to enjoy immediately afterward, as the ritual of sharing it makes the transition back into the mundane world more gradual and pleasant. Touch is very important at this point. Allow for reentry (no pun intended) to take as long as it takes for you both to feel comfortable.

As noted earlier, if you go on to have anal intercourse, it's important to use condoms to prevent transmission of HIV or other STDs. There's a very real danger here, because a great deal of Crisco can remain in an ass and cause a condom to fail very quickly, and condoms are *much* thinner than gloves. Fisting expands the anal tissue, creating microscopic tears or surface abrasions that can provide entry points for semen or pre-come.

After you've been fisted, give your anal passage a break for at least a couple of days so that it can recover. Do *not* douche, as it may irritate your system. Your rectum will expel any residual lube in its own time. Your bowel movements should return within a day; don't be surprised if the initial ones are coated with a bit of lube or mucosal lining. If you feel any residual cramping, rumbling, or other gas pain, you can try the techniques described in Chapter Four, "Hygiene and Diet," in the section titled "Avoiding and Dealing with Gas." Otherwise, gas pain should resolve itself within a day, along with any soreness or slight spotting of blood. On the rare chance that you have more severe symptoms such as a fever, intense pain, or more than slight bleeding, please see a doctor as soon as possible.

Black, tarry stools are a sign of significant internal bleeding. If this occurs, go to the emergency room right away and be honest about how you were injured—your life may depend on it.

## Way Beyond

Some of us have seen or heard of fisters who go all the way up to the elbow or even further into their partner. To many, achieving this kind of deep penetration seems like a magic trick, dangerous as hell, or both.

### Why Would Someone Do That?

Well, because they can. People climb mountains because they're there to be climbed. We attempt difficult things to experience the thrill of exhilaration when we achieve our goal. Being penetrated so deeply requires breaching the barrier between the rectum and the descending colon ("the second hole"). Fisters who experience this say that it's just as thrilling as being fisted for the first time.

### How Do They *Do* That?

Opening up the second hole takes determination, practice, and huge amounts of patience, just like opening the ass in the first place. All of the techniques outlined above in the section "Some Tips and Tricks" apply here as well. Additional specialized techniques can be applied for successful second-hole play. These techniques involve toys and fingers.

## Toys

Playing with long dildos, either as part of solo play or as part of your scene with your partner, is one means of penetrating the second hole. You'll probably want to be on your back when you do this; a sling is ideal. There's some degree of controversy as to whether it's best to use these toys alone or with a partner. One school of opinion has it that an extra pair of hands to guide the toy may come in, well, *handy*. Another school of thought says that in the early stages of opening one's ass deeply, it's absolutely critical that you be the one driving, to control exactly the amount of direction and the pressure of the toy. I recommend that you discuss this with someone experienced in this specialty before proceeding.

Width isn't as important as length; ideally, you want a dildo that's about a foot and a half long. You (or your partner) can line up your intestinal tract to receive a straight object by pushing down once you're inside.

If you're even contemplating this advanced stage of butt play, I hope you know not to use anything except a toy designed for this purpose. A double-headed dildo may do the trick. If your neighborhood adult bookstore doesn't stock toys that are long enough, I recommend one of the vendors in Chapter Fourteen, "Resources," such as Mercury Mail Order or Mr. S.

## Fingers

Whenever you play with a partner, have them enter you "fingers first" rather than using a clenched fist. Your partner should be able to find your second hole with his or her fingertips. If you're comfortable with taking a fist, your partner should be able to work a finger or two, or even three, into your second hole if they're gentle.

The second hole is highly reactive and can close down quickly. When this happens, the entire passage shuts down as well. Thus, you should leave fingering the second hole until the end of your play.

After a few weeks or months of toys and fingers, your second hole will probably be hungry for more active play. Have the inserter go deeper during any handball play. Gradually it will be easier for them to insert more fingers through your second hole. When this happens, you'll be almost ready to take a whole fist through your second hole. Review "Some Tips and Tricks" above, particularly the tip on crunching into a U shape. When you're on the verge of taking the fist past the second hole, one good, slow crunch will often do the trick.

NOTES

1. R. A. Fournier, "The Intelligent Man's Guide to Handball (the sexual sport)," as quoted on the website Redright, www.winternet.com/~redright/redright.html, 1983. See Chapter Fourteen, "Resources," for urls.

2. A respected supplier for these stand-alone units is JIM Support at http://jimsupportportasling.homestead.com/portasling.html. See Chapter Fourteen "Resources," for details, including complete contact information.

3. R. A. Fournier, material in this paragraph reprinted.

# 11

# Extreme Sex: S/M, Gender Play, Fetishes, Piss Play, and Scat Play

*Sometimes I love to get dominated when I'm bottoming. As a young person, I really wasn't in control of things, and as I became an adult, the various professions I've been in have been ones where I have to be in total control or people can get hurt. To totally get dominated by somebody is such a thrill. The vulnerability—a lot of times, I don't like to admit when I can be vulnerable. It's scary, but it's really good.*

## S/M and Anal Play

Some people find it highly erotic to assume control over or surrender control to another in a sexual context. This is what happens in *domination and submission (D/S* for short). When pain is used as a component of this control, we refer to this as *sadomasochism (S/M)*.

In both D/S and S/M, the *top* is generally the doer, and the *bottom* is generally the one to whom things are done. There are many exceptions to this, such as the top ordering the bottom to perform cunnilingus, fellatio, or analingus, but generally, the top sets the agenda during play and the bottom controls the limits of that play.

A wide range of activities fall under the S/M banner, including but not limited to role-playing (for example, master/slave, daddy/girl, coach/athlete, jailer/prisoner), bondage (rope, shackles, cages, temporary mummification), impact (spanking, whipping, caning, paddling, slapping), body modification (cutting, piercing, branding, corseting), and sensory deprivation (blindfolds, hoods, earplugs, gags, breath control). Most of these activities can be combined with anal sex.

S/M can involve intense stimulation at or near the edge of pleasure and pain ("pleasure/pain," sometimes rethought as "sensation play"), the desire to humiliate or be humiliated ("humiliation play"), or both in varying combinations. It's quite possible to influence or effect a mental state using S/M. By using the imagination (and perhaps a blindfold), one can convince a partner or oneself that a certain feeling or activity is taking place when in fact it's not, or convince oneself that the feeling or activity is more extreme or intense than it actually is. Likewise, the feelings of vulnerability that most of us associate with anal receptivity can be amplified using S/M.

Because anal sex is already a taboo activity in our culture, it's easy to exploit that taboo for erotic pleasure, using humiliation, pleasure/pain, or both. However, incorporating the pleasure/pain boundary with anal stimulation carries the potential for physical harm. To play safely with this boundary, it's important to be observant enough to gauge whether something is risky or safe. It's vital that players know the difference between fantasy, pain that's manageable, and pain that has the potential for real damage. This is one reason that *negotiation*[1] (described below) is an important part of S/M anal play.

Many people fantasize about intense or even brutal S/M in conjunction with anal sex but find it too scary to actualize their fantasies. If this is the case for you, then it's important to give yourself permission to enjoy the fantasy but seek sexual satisfaction in other ways. There's nothing wrong with having a fantasy life containing elements that you never actualize, and in many cases it's far preferable (such as with rape or unprotected anal sex). Thinking and doing are very different things.

The world is full of psychically wounded, emotionally damaged people with unresolved issues, some of whom look to the S/M community as a place to act out their frustration in unhealthy ways. Thus, you should use at least as much discretion in selecting a partner for S/M play as you would for any kind of anal play. In the S/M community, reputation is coin of the realm. Anyone who has been around the S/M community for a while will have some sort of "track record" as a player. If you have any doubts at all about a prospective partner, ask them who they have played with, what they did, and how it went. If you know someone whom your potential partner has played with, ask if they'll tell you a bit about how it went.

## Negotiation

Determining with a partner what direction an S/M scene will take requires *negotiation*. This is where turn-ons and turn-offs, physical limitations, and emotional boundaries are discussed. Codified by the erotic underground, sexual negotiation is a process that could benefit the "vanilla" mainstream.

As with most aspects of life, negotiation is an imperfect process. There will always be gray areas that aren't completely anticipated—and often it's the unexpected that can make S/M (as well as anal sex!) exciting. It's impossible, of course, to cover every contingency, but it's important for both partners to have a mutual sense of security and comfort before they go leaping off together. In a sense, then, negotiation is the safety net under the trapeze.

- *Consent* means that you and your partner(s) have agreed to engage in a particular activity. Consent can be oral or nonverbal, explicit or implied; often it's just a look or a lack of action to stop an initiated activity. Some people, especially in the initial stages of S/M exploration, will agree to use a safeword, which can be used to slow or stop a scene if it becomes too intense, dangerous, or otherwise threatening.

- *Consensual nonconsensuality* is an agreement between partners that the top has complete control of the scene and its limits. This is best reserved for very experienced players who are quite comfortable with each other. This isn't something to attempt while in the "getting to know you" stage of dating or while on recreational drugs. Consensual nonconsensuality is a component of edge play, a term for S/M play that borders on or involves actual physical or psychological danger.

## Bondage and Anal Play

*My favorite time was with a lawyer over in Oakland. I was bottom then. It was especially hot because it involved a lot of bondage and giving up of power. I guess we were each in the right mood.*

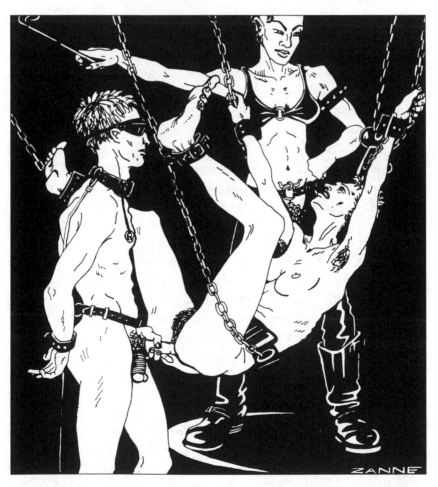

**18. S/M and Anal Sex**

Bondage involves the use of physical restraint. Some considerations when combining bondage and anal play:

- In combining bondage and anal penetration, the top should tie the bottom to allow for any desired access to the anus and rectum; otherwise, the top may have to redo the bondage, or scrap plans altogether. Consider the angle that the bottom's rectum will end up in when the bondage is in place.
- It's important to ensure that breath and blood flow aren't constricted as a result of bondage that's too tight or misplaced.
- Bondage bottoms should never be left unattended.
- In the event of "bondage panic," the bottom should be encouraged to breathe deeply and slowly. It's also helpful for the top to maintain eye contact with the bottom and use a calm tone of voice. On rare occasions, a "button" (emotional trigger) may be pushed accidentally, causing the bottom to lash out in anger. In such cases, it may be safer to leave the bottom in bondage until they have calmed down.
- Obviously, restricting movement is an important aspect of bondage, but how about restricting sight or sound? In any scene, whether it involves bondage, S/M, anal sex, or any combination, blindfolds can heighten physical sensation for the bottom and add to the drama—and prevent the bottom from seeing the top's fumblings, which may be encouraging to a fledgling top!
- Any bondage or anal device should be easy to remove quickly in the event of a problem. This is especially true in any scene in which the bottom may lose control of bodily functions, such as a combination of bondage and enema play. Snub-nosed rope scissors come in handy for quick release from

rope bondage or plastic wrap mummification; check with the vendors listed in Chapter Fourteen, "Resources."

## Fetish Clothing and Other Forms of "Drag"

Underpants and their ilk (jockstraps, crotchless panties, boxers) can be a delightful enhancement to a scene involving butt play of any sort. The garment can stay in place for the duration, or you can find a way to make its eventual removal an erotically charged moment. Pulling down a lover's underpants is an action that many of us find erotic and charged with associations, perhaps as far back as from childhood before a spanking or an enema was administered. You can experiment with removing clothing at a teasing, gradual rate, or a startling, rapid rate. Some folks even like to shred or cut off underwear with a knife or scissors, or perhaps tear a hole in the appropriate spot for anal stimulation. However, you may not want to shred your lover's eighty-dollar silk panties if you haven't checked it out with them first!

Furthermore, don't use any sharp instrument on a lover (or yourself) unless you're fully experienced with it. Check with any S/M organizations that are in your area; they frequently offer workshops on topics such as knife play, bondage, erotic spanking, and dozens of other erotic variations. You can find such groups listed in my own publication, *The Black Book,*[2] as well as in fetish magazines and fetish organization sites online.

Some folks enjoy wearing leather or rubber chaps during anal sex. These provide unlimited access to the genitals and butt; however, they can be a substantial investment. A less expensive alternative to leather (and easier to clean—one friend wears them right into the shower to soap and rinse them off) are the washable chaps available from www.nastypig.com ($150 at this writing; some fetish stores also carry the manufacturer's products).

Don't underestimate the erotic potential of uniforms, either: A construction worker could have all kinds of crazy tools in a tool belt. You can don a nurse's uniform or surgical greens to administer an enema. You can get into role-playing if it works for both of you, or just be yourself and let the suggestiveness of the uniform work its own subtle magic. Let your imagination loose and see what makes you hot.

## Gender Play

Because of the association between anal and vaginal penetration, many men fantasize themselves as women when they're getting fucked, whether by a penis or by a man or woman with a strap-on. Strap-ons enable a woman to be a penetrator, and perhaps to discover a dominant persona. (At this writing, there are two books dedicated to strap-ons; see Chapter Fourteen, "Resources," for details.)

Because of the association between gay men and anal sex, some lesbians and heterosexuals fantasize themselves as gay men while having anal sex. Here's an interesting item, though: According to at least one source, more heterosexual women have done anal than have gay men.[3]

Gender play can be a way to explore assuming a more dominant or submissive role during sex. Gender roles can be fluid, switching back and forth during the course of anal play, or even combining aspects of male and female at the same moment. Gender play can be serious or silly, outrageous or subtle. You might even discover unexplored aspects of yourself and begin to question your assumptions about what's masculine and what's feminine.

Some people find that wearing underpants or other clothing normally associated with the opposite sex heightens their arousal and their fantasies. The same goes for makeup, removable facial hair, rubber masks, or just about anything else that could be used in a typical theatrical setting.

The anus is the great equalizer—after all, everybody has one—so, combined with the right toys and a bit of imagination, anyone can be male or female, dominant or submissive, enacting any number of fantasies in a plethora of configurations of gender roles. Think of gender play as sexual theater.

## Electrical Play

As with enema play, electroplay is a specialized form of sex with a breadth beyond the scope of this book. If you're interested in exploring further, I recommend the book *Juice,* by "Uncle Abdul," published by Greenery Press.

There are a few basics you should know:
- The main thing to know is that the implements made by manufacturers such as Folsom Electric and Paradise Electro Stimulations can be used painfully in an S/M torture context, or pleasurably for stimulating various parts of the body, including the anal canal (usually with a butt plug hooked up to an electric box). There's always controversy about which company's electric box system works better than

another's. I recommend that you do your own research before investing in these expensive toys, by talking to at least two people who actually use them. Contact your local leather shop or sex toy store for further information, as well as any S/M support groups in your area—they may even offer a workshop on electroplay. You can also try a Web search on "electroplay" and contact consumers (perhaps a professional dominant with a Web page) as well as manufacturers.

- All mucosal type tissue is changed (microburns and other effects) by the application of current. No one really knows the consequences of repeated long-term use of electrostimulation to the inside of the body, as applied in play. Therefore, observe the golden rule: "When in doubt, don't do it." The studies that apply to the mode, current levels, and waveforms used are mostly for electrolysis, which involves a different application of current to the body.

- It's possible to design a current using therapeutic, clinical knowledge of mucosal response to electricity, but to my knowledge no one has designed a unit for electroplay using such data.

- Use medical-quality conductive gel and medical grade pads for your connections.

## Piss Play

Also called *golden showers* or *water sports, piss play* involves urination on or in someone (either another person or oneself). Bear in mind a few points:

- As with douching, any butt play tends to stimulate and fill the bladder, so many folks need to pee a lot during play.

- Peeing onto unbroken skin is safe.
- If no virus is being transmitted, piss is sterile. Urine in the kidneys is so close to sterile as to make no difference. Urine in the bladder, though, might have a few dying bacteria wandering about. Urine as it passes through the male urethra picks up a few more bacteria. (As it passes through the shorter female urethra, it picks up fewer.) If urine has enough bacteria to culture or find in a low-strength microscope, there's likely a problem.
- Sharing piss can transmit medications and recreational drugs that aren't processed by the liver, as well as some viruses. Ingesting urine is considered a low-risk activity for transmission of HIV. However, if you're on medication (for HIV or any other condition) and want to engage in this kind of play, I advise you to find a kink-friendly (or at least nonjudgmental) doctor if at all possible. True, doctors don't have all the answers, but those who deal with sexual subcultures may be able to help answer your questions about piss play (such as relative safety and timing of dosage), or can steer you toward other useful resources.
- Carbon dioxide opens up the kidneys. To increase your volume of piss during play, you don't have to drink beer; you can drink soda water or any carbonated drink for the same increase. Increased volume also means more dilute urine, which tends to be weaker-tasting (and hence more palatable to those who like to swallow piss).
- Some people like to share piss (orally or anally) by urinating into a container such as a glass or enema bag, then feeding it to the recipient via a tube.
- Some people like to put their own piss into their butts using an enema. Others prefer to drink their own

piss. It's possible, though unlikely, that folks who play this way can create an autoimmune condition for themselves, leading to health complications.

• As with every other fetish, there are support groups both online and in the real world, together with a mind-boggling array of subspecialties. I suggest that you hook up with long-time players if this sort of play interests you.

## Scat Play

The eroticization of the defecation process, or its by-product (feces, stool, shit, turds), is termed *scat play*. Whether you're interested in this form of erotic play or not, it's important to acknowledge that shit can appear occasionally and unintentionally during most forms of anal play, and you should be psychologically and logistically prepared for it.

Nowadays the Internet is one place to find information and resources on scat play; I provide a short list in Chapter Fourteen, "Resources," for interested readers. Elimination can be a highly pleasurable experience in its own right. Many people experience a quiet joy when they eliminate—it feels good, both physiologically and psychologically. The elimination process often stimulates the same rich network of anal-ring nerve endings that are pleasurable to stimulate during anal play. Relieving the internal pressure also feels good and can produce a sense of peace and relaxation. Some find sharing this normally solitary moment to be highly erotic and intimate. Also, elimination is enjoyable because it marks a completion, and because it's satisfying to pass a well-formed stool. Many of us even secretly enjoy looking at our "creations" before we flush them away.

There's nothing wrong or perverse about being pleased with or interested in one's bodily functions. They're just as much a part of the miracle of life as any other. In fact, as children, we tend to experience this awe quite readily until our curiosity is discouraged.

Some people find scat play to be the ultimate form of intimacy, since it involves an acceptance of their own or their partner's entirety, even those parts that we typically might find repulsive. Also, scat play is sometimes used in erotic domination scenarios to demonstrate one person's profound degree of power over another.

But is it unnatural or perverted? Well, those are subjective terms that have no absolute definition. Many believe any form of anal sex at all to be unnatural and perverted. In a literal sense, however, you could say that the only unnatural sexual act is the one that no one can do. Some men can suck their own penises whereas others can't. Does this make it unnatural?

Scat play can be solo, coupled, or in a group setting. There's a wide range of activities within this category. Roughly by degree of contact, they are: voyeurism (watching someone expel a turd), smell (some individuals find erotic the smell of a lover's shit), touch (eliminating on someone else's body, touching or taking someone's feces from their anal cavity, playing with one's own feces, or smearing feces on one's own body), and ingestion (licking/chewing/swallowing).

Playing with scat can be safe if the play is limited to nonmucosal surfaces, that is, intact skin, since the skin is a highly protective barrier against germs. If you get it on your hands, be careful not to touch your eyes, nose, mouth, anus, vagina, tip of the penis, or any broken skin, otherwise you'll risk germ infection. Thorough washing will kill germs: Use an antibacterial soap such as Dial Liquid, one of the antibacterial dish-washing detergents, or Hibiclens or Betadine.

Ingestion is the most risky of the above activities. Unless you know your partner's complete health history (and even when you do), you may be playing with fire. However, there are ways to reduce harm, such as taking antioxidant vitamins and acidophilus supplements before and after play. Also, avoid excessive douching, which can wipe out the "good" bacteria in your intestines and make it harder to fight off infections and the "bad" bacteria that the body could normally handle.

Most of the bacteria present in feces don't cause disease in humans, but if any disease-causing germs (pathogens) are present, then ingestion is highly danger-ous. Unfortunately, certain bacteria that would otherwise not cause disease will do so when a large enough quan-tity of infectious material is ingested orally or rectally.

If you take stool in your mouth or rectum, you open yourself up to any infectious agent that can be transmit-ted by stool—namely, bacteria, viruses, and parasites. (See Chapter Thirteen, "Anal Health," for a discussion of these.) Most of these pathogens are transmitted by the "fecal–oral route" and aren't as likely to be encountered in other forms of anal play, although since fisters may indirectly come into contact with stool, they can trans-mit such pathogens to themselves if they aren't cautious during play (for example, by wiping an eye with a hand, and other inadvertent contact).

**Health-Related Issues**

RISKS

Hepatitis, intestinal parasites, and other STDs, including HIV, can be communicated via feces. The fecal–oral route is the main mode of transmission of most hepatitis viruses, particularly hepatitis B.[4] (By the way, you can be a carrier for hepatitis and not know it; your health care provider can test you for this.) Even with an HIV-negative partner, when you ingest someone else's feces, in essence you're taking into your own system their intestinal flora, the balance of good and bad bugs that's unique to each person. Doing this could profoundly throw off your body's balance. Finally, the medications and treatments for these pathogens (such as Flagyl or Cipro for parasites) can be difficult for some to handle as well.

PRECAUTIONS

You can have yourself inoculated against hepatitis A and B, but not yet C. (Further details are included in Chapter Thirteen, "Anal Health.") Also, it's advisable for folks into scat play to have themselves vaccinated against the flu every fall and to have the pneumonia vaccine as well.

It would be wise to have both partners' stools tested for infection. Have a stool culture and sensitivity, ova, and parasite test. Note that problems are not always detected in stool samples—for instance, giardia lives in the intestinal mucosa (the inner lining), not in the stool itself—and you'll have to submit several samples to be reasonably safe. If you're into this play, then it's a good idea to have your stool tested on a regular basis anyhow. Typically, your health professional will run the "routine screen," which doesn't cover all possible infections or parasites. You probably don't have to give him or her all the details regarding your scat play, but you can say that you're having sex with other men (even if your scat play is exclusively with women) and want to be checked for some of the infections that gay men can transmit. (One possible scenario, a euphemistic possibility for shy patients, is to explain that you've played with rimming, which will cause them to run the same sorts of tests they'd run if you'd said you were into scat.) Another possibility is to get a testing referral to the "tropical diseases" specialist or department at your hospital.

Some scat enthusiasts recommend regular consumption of acidophilus capsules as a way to ensure that the "good bugs" are ever-present in your system, as well as a prophylaxis measure against many dangerous ones. You can get these at a natural foods store. The refrigerated kind are the best, I'm told. Yogurt and acidophilus milk may help too.

## FECES AND FISTING

If significant amounts of feces are present during fisting, the mucosa of the rectum and colon could break down, allowing bacteria to enter the deeper layers of the colon, creating an abscess, or entering even further, reaching the abdominal cavity to cause peritonitis, which can be deadly. Many people with normal diets eat certain foods that don't break down even in the rectum, such as particles of nuts, corn, and other foods that are indigestible to humans. These particles can act as irritants and cause breaks in the mucosa.

## SELF-PLAY

Can you infect yourself by playing with or eating your own shit? Not literally, but doing so can still have serious health consequences. Your stool is waste material discarded by the body and is identified by your body as such.

If you're concerned about this, discuss it with your health care provider and have him or her check that you haven't started an autoimmune process. If you are uncomfortable discussing this or any other scat-related issue with your physician, you can try finding a suitable professional through the Kink Aware Professionals list at www.bannon.com/kap or by checking the scat-play references in Chapter Fourteen, "Resources."

## Combining Fetishes

> *For countless thousands of people all over this world, enemas and spankings go hand in hand.*
> —DAVID BARTON-JAY, THE ENEMA AS AN EROTIC ART AND ITS HISTORY[5]

If you can think about a particular sexual act or combination of acts, it's near-certain that someone else has recently done it, is doing it now, or is thinking about doing it soon.

The Internet has made it easier for folks interested in esoteric fetishes or unusual combinations of fetishes to find each other. See Chapter Fourteen, "Resources," for a list of some places you can start.

> *To some people, the idea of having someone administer an enema is exciting. For them the sensation of the water inside seems like an extension of being flooded with come.*
> —DR. CHARLES SILVERSTEIN AND EDMUND WHITE, THE JOY OF GAY SEX

Enema play seems to combine particularly well with other forms of fetish, such as bondage, spanking, shaving, and role-playing. "Teenage Enema Nurses in Bondage" was the title of a Punk-era song by Killer Pussy that I still hear occasionally. That rather says it all.

## NOTES

1.  The credo of the S/M community is "safe, sane, and consensual." *Safe* means that the partners are using reasonable precautions to ensure that the scene isn't physically or mentally damaging. *Sane* means that neither partner is too drunk, drugged, or mentally unstable to play responsibly. *Consensual* means that both partners have negotiated and agreed to the limits and general outline of the scene.

2.  *The Black Book*, published by Black Books, (800) 818-8823.

3.  *Homosexualities*, by Martin Weinberg and Clive Bell (1979).

4.  www.pigmedia.com/health.htm#scat

5.  David Barton-Jay, *The Enema as an Erotic Art and Its History* (The David Barton-Jay Projects, P.O. Box 1235, Brattleboro, VT 05302, 1996).

# 12

# Recreational Drugs and Sex

I am providing this information about drugs most commonly used in conjunction with sex so that you can make rational, safer, and informed decisions about drug use. I'm not endorsing the use of illegal substances. If you don't use illegal substances, I am not recommending that you start. If you do use them, I hope you find this information useful. Neither I nor the publisher will be held liable for any misunderstanding or misuse of information provided herein. If you have further questions, please consult the support resources listed in Chapter Fourteen.

A few important points about drugs in general:

- Recreational drugs impair your judgment to some extent for varying lengths of time and increase the risk of unsafe sex.

- Drugs tend to make people sloppy and careless, which may be part of the attraction—but this can also increase the risk of unsafe sex.
- Many people use a variety of recreational drugs over the course of their lives with no apparent ill effects.
- Any damage to the human body on a regular basis, such as through drug use, is cumulative.
- If you do use drugs, don't have an agenda. You can damage yourself more readily by trying to do too much, too fast. Combining extreme anal play with recreational drugs increases this likelihood.
- Your drug experiences will be more meaningful and memorable if you reserve drugs for special occasions and treat them as a "sacrament" you're only willing to share with loved ones you feel comfortable with. You'll also be less likely to get yourself into dangerous situations if you're on drugs with people whom you trust.

## Alcohol

Most of us know the effects and risks of using alcohol, so I'll limit my words to a few essential points.

- Alcohol profoundly impairs judgment, which makes risky behavior more likely.
- Alcohol reduces your sharpness of perception, which makes accidents more likely.
- Drinking too much alcohol (more than one or two servings) may make you unable to get a hard-on.
- It's a bad idea to consume alcohol in conjunction with any medications, such as HIV drugs, where it is contraindicated.
- Alcohol dehydrates you, so drink plenty of water and fluids to replenish the lost body fluids.

- Raw alcohol should never be given as an enema, as it can damage your internal organs. The body processes alcohol through the liver, so consuming it rectally circumvents this process! The mucosa absorbs the alcohol even more quickly than the body does when you sip a drink, which means that rectally you'll get really drunk really fast and perhaps poison yourself.

  Experiencing a light buzz by putting a couple of teaspoons of wine in a regular enema is probably OK for most people, but please be extremely careful and don't ever use more than a tablespoon total. Always give your body at least a week to recover and heal before doing this again.

## Cocaine

While alcohol is a depressant, cocaine is a stimulant, meaning that it gets you up and keeps you going. Unlike speed (a synthetic stimulant described below), cocaine is a natural extract from the leaf of the coca bush.

When cocaine enters the body, it moves rapidly to the central nervous system where it acts on the reward/pleasure centers of the brain, which produce an important pleasure chemical, *dopamine*. These parts of your brain aid with thought organization, concentration, fine motor control, sex drive, and energy. Initially, cocaine increases all these functions. However, as cocaine use increases, the brain's natural receptor sites reduce or even lose their ability to produce these chemicals, which causes feelings of depression or a "crash."

Other bodily responses include increased heart rate, blood pressure, and breathing rate. Cocaine also increases alertness, stamina, and feelings of euphoria while reducing fatigue, the desire to sleep, and hunger.

Cocaine sold on the street is cut with various substances to increase profits, including lactose (a diuretic), procaine (a local anesthetic that makes you lose feeling), and other drugs.

Snorting cocaine causes nasal damage by deteriorating the mucosa of the cartilage in the nose. Long-term use may eat a hole through your septum.

Smoking cocaine can result in throat and lung damage, stroke, abnormal heart rhythms, and extremely high blood pressure. It can result in cut lips (especially smoking with a broken glass stem), which increases the risk of contracting HIV, hepatitis, and other infectious diseases. Sharing pipes or stems can transmit herpes and tuberculosis as well. If you smoke cocaine, cover the mouthpiece with rubber or tape to prevent cuts or heat burns.

Most people experience an intense crash after cocaine use that can include physical exhaustion, cold-like symptoms, depression, and anxiety.

As with all recreational drugs, eat, sleep, and drink plenty of water and juice, even if you're not hungry and especially if you've been on a binge.

## Ecstasy

MDMA, popularly known as "ecstasy" or simply "E" or "X," is a synthetic, psychoactive (mind-altering) "designer drug" with hallucinogenic and amphetamine-like properties. Its chemical composition is similar to that of two other synthetic drugs, MDA and methamphetamine, which are known to cause brain damage.

Ecstasy works by increasing your body's level of serotonin. Serotonin is a brain substance that controls your emotions. When you have more of it, you may feel more emotional and trusting of others, experiencing "universal love." X is sometimes called "the love drug." The duration of the peak experience is about 90 minutes.

Typically, ecstasy comes in pill or capsule form. It takes about 30 minutes for the user to start feeling its effects. You peak in about 90 minutes, and it wears off after three or four hours. As with other "street drugs," you never really know what you're getting when you buy ecstasy; it may contain other drugs like LSD, speed, or K (ketamine).

Disappointingly, most users never fully recapture the magic of their first few trips. Moreover, X may even be harmful at subtherapeutic doses. As the uncertain process of neural recovery sets in, heavy users in particular may experience the subtle, drawn-out reversal of all the positive feelings they initially experienced from the drug.

Dancing on X can cause dehydration due to sweating, which can lead to heart attacks or strokes, even in young people. Signs of dehydration include muscle cramping, disoriented feelings, and feverish sensations with no sweat. If you use X, be sure to drink plenty of water afterward.

Ecstasy may indirectly cause the spread of HIV, hepatitis, and other STDs because users may have sex without taking normal precautions. Always have condoms on hand, and insist on using them!

Many problems that users encounter with MDMA are similar to those found with the use of amphetamines and cocaine. They are:

- Psychological difficulties, including confusion, depression, sleep difficulty, drug craving, severe anxiety, and paranoia, both during and sometimes weeks after taking ecstasy. In rare cases, psychotic episodes have been reported.

- Physical symptoms, such as muscle tension, involuntary teeth-clenching, nausea, blurred vision, rapid eye movements, faintness, and chills or sweating.
- Increases in heart rate and blood pressure, a special risk for people with circulatory or heart disease.

## Marijuana

People react differently to pot. Some folks find it relaxes them while others find that it makes them "hyper" and keeps them up late. The variety of marijuana can affect the type of high, but don't assume that you and your partner will have the same reaction to it.

Some people become very talkative on pot, which may reduce their ability to focus on sex. Marijuana can induce paranoia (particularly among proponents of "The War on Drugs"!). More typically, though, it leaves the user pleasantly and harmlessly stoned. Users may experience sleepiness, euphoria, and pain relief. As with other hallucinogens (such as "magic" mushrooms), euphoria, excitement, and inner happiness—often accompanied by hilarity and laughter—are typical. Pot may also cause users to feel less physically inhibited, which explains its popularity as an aphrodisiac.

It can also induce feelings of apathy and an impairment of cognitive function, albeit moderately and reversibly. Marijuana interferes with memory formation by disrupting long-term potentiation in the hippocampus, a brain region that's believed to play an important role in certain forms of learning and memory. This may explain the short-term amnesia or "spaciness" that many users experience. Forgetting is not, as one might assume, a purely passive process. Choosing deliberately to ingest an amnesiac agent over a long period of time is scarcely an ideal life-strategy. It's especially flawed, given the centrality of memory to human self-identity.

It's very important to drink lots of water before, during, and after taking pot, whether it's smoked or eaten. Some people get chilled from taking marijuana, so it's important that your playspace be well-heated and that you have ready access to blankets or bedding to take away the chill. Some find that taking pot reduces blood flow to and sensation in the extremities, which may be a physical distraction that impinges on their enjoyment of sex.

## Poppers

Amyl or butyl nitrite, also known as poppers, are perhaps the most commonly used recreational drug for anal sex, particularly among gay and bisexual men. Poppers give you a rush—a near-immediate speeding up of the pulse—and a sudden lightheadedness that lasts up to several minutes. This is primarily the result of oxygen deprivation to the brain. Users find these sensations pleasurable in combination with sex, where they're used to make anal penetration easier and to intensify orgasm. Poppers reduce blood build-up and cause a drop in blood pressure because they relax the smooth muscles of the vascular system. Some people find that, as a result of these changes, poppers relax the anal sphincters. They also give some users a headache.

Poppers are available via mail order and in some of the places that sell leather goods, porn videotapes, and sex toys. Often you need to use the correct "code word" to gain access. Poppers are sold variously as video head cleaner, leather cleaner, carburetor cleaner, solvent, and so forth. Quality varies widely, and some brands contain unknown, potentially toxic ingredients.

An occasional sniff of poppers is probably not going to hurt you. The problem, as with other drugs used for sex, is that for many of us, it's hard to limit usage to an occasional dose. While it's unlikely that poppers are physically addictive, with repeated use, they can become psychologically addictive to the point where some users don't find sex satisfying without them.

Don't use poppers at all when you're taking Viagra; both cause a drop in blood pressure, and combining them can cause loss of consciousness, even strokes.

If you use poppers, be extremely careful not to tip the bottle back too far, which is easy when you're lying on your back or in a sling. (To prevent this, you may want to get an inhaler, a bullet-shaped device made of aluminum.) If you spill this stuff, it's nasty. First, it's going to blow your scene. Get up immediately and blot away any that has spilled on your skin. Next, wash it off your skin with soap and warm water. If you spill it in your nose, gently blow out any residual liquid. It will probably sting, and you will probably feel very disoriented for a little while. Stay calm.

It amazes me how many fisters and others into anal sex will get their hands all greasy and then attempt to handle this small, slippery glass bottle that has no flow control, is a dark color (to help prevent deterioration from light), has a removable black lid, making it hard to see, and expect not to spill it. (By the way, if you happen to smear grease on the rim of or inside the bottle, your poppers' potency will deteriorate rapidly.)

As an aside, I've seen men who made love to their little brown bottle more attentively than to their sex partners.

If you're going to use poppers, take a couple of pre-cautions to help protect yourself. Take a two-gram dose of vitamin C a bit before using poppers, if possible, and another afterward. This will reduce the concentration of immunity-compromising free radicals in your system. Also, drinking plenty of water before, during, and after play is always a good idea, even if you don't do drugs, but especially if you do. Consistent hydration appears to reduce the negative effects of any drug hangover.

A common question is whether poppers are immunosuppressive. One brochure claims: "Your immune response dips immediately on inhaling poppers, and stays down for about 96 hours. An already compromised immune system [as with HIV] can suffer even more damage from repeated popper use." It says further that "dilated blood vessels in the rectum make it easier for viruses and other germs to enter your blood stream." Finally, it states that "use of poppers in enclosed areas can have a negative effect on HIV+ people breathing the [secondhand fumes]."[1] Also, poppers may reduce the effectiveness of HIV drugs. On the other hand, there's no apparent permanent damage. A kink-sensitive health professional asserts in an Internet FAQ: "There were many studies of this during the 1980s at the center where I trained, New York University. Poppers [per se] do not lower your white cell count or make you more likely to get HIV or (as was once thought) give you AIDS."[2]

## Methamphetamine
### (a/k/a Speed, Crystal, Tina, Crank)

Speed is a synthetic stimulant. It affects your central nervous system in the same way that adrenaline (your body's natural stimulant) works. The short-term effects on the nervous system are pretty much identical to those of cocaine (although far more prolonged), so you can read about those in the cocaine section, above.

Dopamine is the "pleasure chemical" in the brain most affected by speed. Speed initially increases the functioning of central nervous system functions and the production of dopamine, creating the high. Eventually, the brain's natural receptor sites stop producing dopamine, and you need the speed to feel good again.

Methamphetamine is a powerful stimulant that's highly addictive. It's often manufactured illegally in underground labs. It's also known as "speed," "Tina," or "crystal" when it's swallowed, sniffed, smoked, or injected, and sometimes as "crank" or "ice." All forms induce long-lasting, debilitating effects.[3]

Methamphetamine sends a message to brain cells to fire more dopamine, a feel-good chemical that's also critical to normal brain functioning. Hours after it's ingested, cell receptors begin to turn off to slow the flow of dopamine, and here's where methamphetamine differs from other stimulants, such as cocaine. While other stimulants allow brain cells to capture and repackage the dopamine, methamphetamine doesn't. The brain cells respond by releasing an enzyme to knock out the extra dopamine. With repeated use, those enzymes eventually kill the dopamine cell, and that leads to a chemical change in the way your brain works.[4]

Methamphetamine can be smoked, injected intravenously, snorted, or ingested orally. The drug alters mood in different ways, depending on how it's taken. Immediately after smoking or intravenous injection, the user experiences an intense "rush" or "flash" that lasts only a few minutes and is described as extremely pleasurable. Smoking or injecting produces effects fastest, within 5 to 10 seconds. Snorting or ingesting orally produces euphoria—a high but not an intense rush. Snorting produces effects within 3 to 5 minutes, and ingesting orally produces effects within 15 to 20 minutes.[5]

The most frequently reported behavioral and psychiatric symptoms include violent behavior, repetitive activity, memory loss, paranoia, delusions of reference, auditory hallucinations, and confusion or fright. Abnormal weight loss is common among repetitive users.[6]

The stimulant effects from methamphetamine can last for hours, instead of minutes as with crack cocaine. Often the methamphetamine user remains awake for days. As the high begins to wear off, the methamphetamine user enters a stage called "tweaking," in which he or she is prone to violence, delusions, and paranoia.[7] One of the most significant dangers with methamphetamine, as opposed to some of the other drugs in this survey, is the user's tendency to binge on the drug. Binges can last up to a week or even longer. Repeated use of methamphetamine rapidly produces strong psychological dependence and a withdrawal syndrome consistent with physical dependence.[8]

Some food for thought on speed use and anal sex:

• Speed is highly compromising to the immune system.
• Speed makes the receiver oblivious to pain. Most serious injury to handballers is associated with methamphetamine use. Tops using it aren't safe for their bottoms either.
• Ongoing speed use significantly rots the teeth, which can result in malnutrition. Malnutrition weakens the immune system. Bleeding gums provide yet another point of entry to HIV, bacteria, and other pathogens during sex.[9]

Don't believe that your body doesn't need to sleep or eat. Eat well and drink lots of water. Minimize alcohol intake, because it also dehydrates you and can lead to a more severe crash. When your trip is over, give your body all the sleep it needs to recover.

If you share syringes, stems, or other paraphernalia to take speed, you're at increased risk for HIV, hepatitis, TB, and other infectious diseases. Use your own paraphernalia and keep them cleaned.

## NOTES

1. "Poppers: Can You Afford the Risk?," disseminated in 1999 via New Leaf, San Francisco.

2. www.pigmedia.com/health.htm

3. www.mninter.net/~publish/Photo47b.htm

4. www.whitehousedrugpolicy.gov/drugfact/methamphetamine/index.html

5. www.nida.nih.gov/NIDA_Notes/NNVol11N5/Tearoff.html

6. Miller, M. A. Trends and patterns of methamphetamine smoking in Hawaii. In: *Methamphetamine Abuse: Epidemiologic Issues and Implications*. M. A. Miller and N. J. Kozel, eds. Rockville, Md.: U.S. Department of Health and Human Services, National Institutes of Health, National Institute on Drug Abuse, June 1995. NIH publication no. 95-3990. National Institute on Drug Abuse, 991. Research monograph 115, DHHS publication no. (AM) 91-1836. Found on www.ctclearinghouse.org/vfmeth.htm

7. Ibid., endnote 4.

8. Ibid.

9. Adapted from www.sexuality.org/l/sex/handball.html, "Handballing Guide" (from a pamphlet published by *Trust Handballing Newsletter*, date unknown, probably early 1990s).

# Anal Health

For most of us, there's no such thing as totally safe sex. I prefer the term *safer sex* because it's more accurate; virtually all sex can have some form of consequence, ranging from emotional risk to pregnancy to disease. Even the experts often disagree on what is and isn't "safe" from a physical health perspective. However, we can realistically assess our own sexual patterns for risk factors and discuss with our sex partners our options for risk management. Starting with a good knowledge of the facts helps us make rational decisions.

If you choose to practice safer sex, then I advise safer sex practices during foreplay as well as intercourse. As soon as you anticipate any contact between the penis and the anal region, put a condom on the penis. Although it's rare for HIV to be spread without ejaculation, pre-come does contain the virus, there can be microscopic tears in the skin, and many other sexually transmitted diseases and conditions *(STDs)* can be spread from skin-to-skin contact (that is, rubbing but not penetrating the anal region): *herpes, gonorrhea, syphilis, anal warts,* and *molluscum.*

## Dealing with Doctors

It's essential to find a doctor with whom you can speak frankly about your sexual history and practices. I highly recommend *Health Care Without Shame* by Dr. Charles Moser,[1] for advice on finding a sex-positive doctor. Race Bannon maintains a listing of Kink Aware Professionals, including physicians and other health care providers.[2]

You might also try dealing with public health department doctors, who tend to be less moralistic and more helpful than many MDs.

It's easy to forget questions and concerns when you're seeing a doctor. Make a list of these and take it with you to the appointment. Do research online or in books before your doctor's appointment.

All adolescents in the United States have the right to diagnosis and treatment of STDs without the consent or knowledge of their parents.[3]

## Anal Irritations

### Anal Itching

Skin around the anus often appears red and cracked and may become callused. Scabs and cuts can appear from scratching during sleep, when itching is usually intensified. Anal itching is usually caused by chronic skin irritation, often an allergy that suddenly develops. Scents found in bath soap, laundry detergent, perfume, or other sources can be the source of contact. Foods, particularly spicy foods, can also irritate the anus when expelled in the stool. The best way to treat anal itching is to determine what has caused the irritation and to eliminate it.

- Change your bath and laundry detergents, as well as any other substances that come into contact with your anal region, such as lubes, massage oils, creams, and lotions.

- Avoid toilet paper, which can be scratchy and irritating. Many contain perfumes and bleaches. Instead, use medicated wipes such as Tucks or cotton balls moistened with witch hazel, or a clean, damp washcloth. Gently wipe or blot the area dry. You can follow this with a thin layer of Balneol lotion. Read labels and avoid using anything on your anus that contains alcohol or perfume.

- Eliminate all potentially irritating foods. These include spicy foods (pepper, garlic, and so on); highly acidic foods and their juices (citrus, tomato, grape, cranberry, and the like) as well as high doses of vitamin C (ascorbic acid); alcohol (including wine); milk products (lactose-free milk or yogurt are exceptions); and anything containing caffeine (coffee, tea, chocolate, and many sodas). Become an expert at reading food labels for suspect ingredients while shopping, and be especially careful when dining out—ask about ingredients used in prepared foods.

- After a month or so, your itching should disappear or be greatly reduced. Then you can try adding back the foods one at a time until you discover the offending ingredient.

### Hemorrhoids

Inflamed, abnormally dilated veins at the end of the rectal canal are called *hemorrhoids*. Normally, the veins act as cushions for the passage of stool. There are two types of hemorrhoids: internal and external. *Internal hemorrhoids* originate inside the rectum but frequently hang outside the rectum as they enlarge. *External hemorrhoids* are enlarged veins under the skin next to the anal opening.

Hemorrhoids occur when normal blood flow through a vein becomes clotted. Bearing down to lift, to pass a bowel movement, or to do anything that increases pressure in your anorectal canal increases the likelihood of hemorrhoids. Simply sitting on the toilet for an extended period of time (say, while reading) can cause hemorrhoids. However, they can be triggered by something as simple as a sneeze or cough. So having a hemorrhoid or any other anorectal disorder isn't an indication that you have been having anal sex.

Your doctor can treat an external hemorrhoid with a simple surgical procedure performed in the exam office using local anesthesia. While most hemorrhoids will resolve themselves without surgery, the procedure is advised, in order to prevent a recurrence. When a hemorrhoid recurs, it's likely to be more painful than it was the previous time.

While anal sex doesn't cause internal hemorrhoids, anal sex may irritate them and cause bleeding. They're rarely painful because there are no nerve endings where the hemorrhoid occurs; however, they can bleed when inflamed. Since rectal bleeding can be a symptom of something more serious, such as colon cancer, you should see a doctor when bleeding occurs.

Those who want to have anal sex while hemorrhoids are a problem should go slowly and try lying on the belly while getting fucked. This position decreases blood flow to the clotted veins.

## Treatment of Hemorrhoids

Hard stools *and* diarrhea can irritate hemorrhoids, so avoid laxatives such as Ex-Lax, constipating treatments such as Imodium, and cathartics such as Epsom salts. In treating hemorrhoids, the goal is to achieve soft yet formed stools. There are several ways to do this:

- *Diet.* Water-absorbing plant fiber stays in the intestine, promoting moister stools and thus making bowel movements less traumatic. High-fiber foods include most fruits (such as prunes), vegetables (such as spinach), and unprocessed grains (such as whole-grain breads and bran cereal). Have several servings a day.

- *Fiber supplement.* Commercial supplements such as Metamucil and Citrucel are widely available. Psyllium husk is available at natural food stores. Be sure to drink plenty of water while taking a fiber supplement and increase dosage gradually; otherwise, the fiber will remain dry and therefore be painful to expel.

- *Stool softeners* such as Colace contain a nonabsorbing mineral oil that stays in the digestive tract and mixes with stool so that it expels more easily.

There are several ways to soothe inflamed hemorrhoids:

- *Suppositories and creams* such as Preparation H or Anusol can provide inflammation relief. Use a cream for external hemorrhoids and a suppository or cream with applicator to treat bleeding caused by internal hemorrhoids. An over-the-counter strength of 1% or 1.5% hydrocortisone should soothe most swelling; a 2.5% concentration is available by pre-scription. Glycerin suppositories are useful if the first part of your stool is hard.

- *Sitz baths* are effective because the warm water helps reduce swelling and relaxes the anal sphincter. You don't need to add anything to the tub water; just be sure it isn't too hot.
- *Witch hazel* is often helpful in reducing swelling and irritation. It's the active ingredient in medicated pads such as Tucks; however, you can also buy a bottle at the pharmacy and apply it using folded toilet tissue or cotton pads. You can keep liquid or pads in the refrigerator and apply them cold for additional soothing action.

## Anal Fissures and Fistulas

### Fissures

An anal fissure is a painful tear in the anal lining. With a mirror, you can usually see the fissure right at or just inside the anal opening. Most often, they're the result of a hard bowel movement tearing the lining. Other causes can be trauma from anal intercourse, fingers, or toys. Fissures usually occur in the side of the anus closest to the tail-bone, but they can occur anywhere if caused by sexual trauma. Chronic irritation often causes a small adjacent pile (skin tag), and it's common to mistake the pile as the source of irritation when in fact it's the crater-like fissure.

TREATMENT OF FISSURES
Take a fiber supplement such as psyllium husk and a stool softener such as Colace. Most cases resolve within several days of beginning treatment.

Keep a box of latex gloves near the toilet with some lubricant so that you can cover up anal tears while passing stool. The tears will heal much more quickly using this method since stool is gritty and abrasive and keeps irritating the tear.

Steroid creams may also help fissures heal more quickly. Some contain a topical anesthetic to relieve pain and relax the sphincter. Finally, warm sitz baths should help as well.

If a fissure occurs while having anal sex, stop immediately and avoid further anal manipulation until healing occurs.

### Fistulas

A fistula is a boil-like infection beside the anal opening that burrows into the skin and pops open like a pimple. Again, it's not usually the result of intercourse. Many people ignore fistulas, but they can develop into abscesses if left untreated.

TREATMENT OF FISTULAS
Surgery is considered the best treatment, and subsequent discomfort is usually minimal.

## Sexually Transmitted Diseases and Conditions

More than half of sexually active adults acquire one or more STDs within their lifetime, and over 12 million Americans are infected with an STD every year.[4] While the lion's share of the attention these days still goes to HIV, many other more-common STDs often go ignored. Most of this chapter is devoted to a discussion of these conditions, in alphabetical order below. I have included all common sexually transmitted conditions where anal sex involving men is a significant cofactor. Missing from this discussion are conditions that predominantly concern women (such as trichomonas), or those that aren't anal-sex specific (such as scabies).

## Chlamydia

TRANSMISSION

*Chlamydia* can be transmitted via oral, genital, or anal sex, and possibly via sex toys. Condoms help prevent transmission.

SYMPTOMS

A person with chlamydia may remain symptom-free for their entire life or may start to show symptoms at any time after an infection. Some infected folks experience burning while urinating. A man or woman who becomes infected with chlamydia as a result of receiving anal intercourse may develop a mucosal discharge from the rectum, rectal bleeding, diarrhea, or bowel movement pain.

TREATMENT

Despite its frequency, most health care providers do *not* offer routine testing for chlamydia unless there's an obvious symptom. However, since chlamydia is so often symptom-free, you'll probably need to ask specifically for chlamydia screening. No test for chlamydia is 100% accurate, so you may wish to repeat the test if it comes back negative, particularly if you have symptoms.[5]

Treatment with an antibiotic is the usual method of treatment. Since chlamydia remains in the system for up to a week after initial treatment, it's important to abstain from sex while taking the antibiotic.

## Epididymitis and Prostatitis

*Epididymitis* and *prostatitis infections* occur in men and can be caused by sexually transmitted bacteria such as those that cause chlamydia and gonorrhea, as well as by bacteria that aren't sexually transmitted. *Epididymitis* infects the *epididymus,* which sits above each testicle and whose function is crucial to the maturation of sperm. Infection usually occurs on only one side of the scrotum. *Prostatitis* infects the *prostate,* the walnut-sized organ at the base of the penis that makes fluid which combines with sperm to make semen.

### TRANSMISSION

Epididymitis and prostatitis in younger men are usually sexually transmitted, often through unprotected anal, oral, or genital intercourse. In older men, either usually occurs because of an enlarged prostate, which can lead to incomplete emptying of the bladder and increased risk for urinary tract infections (UTIs).

### SYMPTOMS

*Epididymitis:* scrotal pain, redness, and swelling, only on one side in most cases. Pain may be severe. Burning urination and discharge may occur. *Prostatitis:* infections are usually classified as acute or chronic. Acute infections manifest severe symptoms such as fever, chills, fatigue, difficulty urinating, increased frequency, or inability to urinate. Chronic infections manifest more subtle symptoms or none. Most men experience difficulty and/or dribbling after urinating, and more frequent urination. Sometimes there's a dull pain in the perineum. There may be pain with ejaculation and blood in the semen. Some men have epididymitis and prostatitis concurrently.

TREATMENT

Epididymitis can usually be treated with antibiotics. Bed rest and scrotal elevation help in draining infection from the testicle. Referral to a urologist is indicated for symptoms that persist after three days.

Antibiotic treatment for prostatitis varies, depending on severity and cause. If sexual transmission is believed to be the cause of acute prostatitis, treatments for other bacterial STDs (chlamydia, gonorrhea) should be initiated.[6]

## Gonorrhea

According to some sources, gonorrhea ("clap") is the most common STD worldwide, and the most frequently reported STD in the United States.[7] Gonorrhea thrives in warm, moist places, so it can live in the throat, rectum, penis, or vagina. About one-fifth of men with gonorrhea have it present at more than one site.

TRANSMISSION

The bacteria that cause gonorrhea can be passed easily through sexual contact, such as intercourse, fellatio, anal sex, cunnilingus, and even kissing, although the last is rare. Condoms are the most effective barrier to transmission.

SYMPTOMS

The most common male symptom is a yellowish or greenish discharge from the penis, or such stains appearing on underwear. Urination may be painful and may occur more frequently than usual. In the anus, gonorrhea produces a discharge that may be mistaken for leaking stool. Blood or mucus may appear in stool. Bowel movements may be uncomfortable. Rectal pain and itching may occur. Symptoms usually appear within 2 to 5 days after infection, although it can take up to 30 days. Roughly 10% of infected men and as many as 40% of infected women have no symptoms.[8] Later stages of the infection in men may move into the prostate, seminal vesicles, and epididymis, causing severe pain and fever. Rare cases can lead to septic arthritis. Untreated gonorrhea can lead to sterility.

TREATMENT

Gonorrhea is a bacterial infection and is therefore treated with antibiotics. Any sexual partners you have had within the past sixty days should be notified and treated as well, even if they're symptomless.

- Gonorrhea and syphilis transmit easily.
- They often go undetected; 10% of men and some 20% to 40% of women are symptom-free.
- Gonorrhea is becoming more difficult to treat. (Syphilis, by contrast, is still easily treatable.)

I recommend that you be tested routinely every six months if you're sexually active with multiple partners, particularly anonymous partners.

**Hepatitis**

The disease *hepatitis* means "inflammation of the liver." The liver helps digest food and eliminate toxins and other things foreign to your body, like drugs. A liver that gets too damaged to work properly poses a life-threatening condition. HIV-positive people should be especially careful to avoid contracting hepatitis, since many of the current antiviral medications are toxic to the liver.

## Hepatitis A

### TRANSMISSION

*Hep A* is caused by contact with particles of infected feces. The most common way this happens is through swallowing contaminated food or water. You can also get it from rimming, sharing contaminated toys, or sucking a penis immediately after it has been in someone's butt. It takes very little virus to transmit infection.

### SYMPTOMS AND TREATMENT

Some people have no symptoms, while others may suffer from some combination of nausea, vomiting, jaundice, diarrhea, and an extreme lack of energy. While hep A is active, you can pass the virus to others, even if you're symptomless. Once you recover, you can't spread hep A and, since your immune system develops antibodies, you're immune to getting it again.

Almost everyone infected with hepatitis A recovers without treatment within four to eight weeks. However, supportive treatment includes rest, fluids, antinausea medications, and total abstention from alcohol.

## Hepatitis B

### TRANSMISSION

*Hep B* is spread by unprotected vaginal, anal, or oral sex with an infected person. Unsterilized tattooing or body piercing equipment can transmit it. It can also be spread by sharing infected syringes and related injection equipment, and possibly via shared crack pipes or straws used to snort drugs. Even sharing toothbrushes or razors may cause infection. Pregnant mothers may also pass it to their fetuses.

SYMPTOMS AND TREATMENT

Most people don't display symptoms, but all can infect others. Nausea, jaundice, and diarrhea are the most common symptoms. Abdominal pain and vomiting are possible. Stools may lighten to a clay color, and urine may darken to a brownish color. Most people recover completely within about six months.

Between 5% and 10% of hep B infectees become lifelong carriers; about a third of them develop chronic liver disease, which can lead to cirrhosis and liver cancer. Approximately 1% of people who acquire hep B die of complications.[9]

Plenty of rest is the best treatment for recovering from hep B. There's no treatment for acute infection. Interferon may be effective against chronic infection.

## Hepatitis C

TRANSMISSION

*Hep C* is usually transmitted via blood contact. It can be spread via the same drug paraphernalia as hep B. Nonsterile tattooing and body-piercing equipment can transmit the virus, too. A pregnant mother can pass it to her fetus. It may be possible to get hep C via razors, toothbrushes, and other shared household objects. In a small percentage of cases, it can be transmitted via sexual contact, although not a lot is known yet about this.

SYMPTOMS AND TREATMENT

Most of us don't know when we are infected with hep C. Most often, we discover the infection years later when we get sick and a test for hep C comes back positive. If symptoms do develop, they're usually mild, occurring four to eight weeks after infection: jaundice, nausea, abdominal pain, appetite loss, and fever.

About 80% of infectees never clear the virus out of the system.[10] These chronically infected carriers can continue to infect others. Fatigue is the most common symptom at this stage.

HEPATITIS PREVENTION

Use protection when having sex (condoms, dental dams, and latex gloves), particularly when rimming or having anal sex. Know your partners and their history if you want to rim without a barrier. Wash your hands thoroughly, preferably with antibacterial soap, after fingering someone's anus. If you're a drug user, avoid sharing paraphernalia.

Get vaccinated against hepatitis A and hepatitis B. At this writing, there's at least one experimental vaccine for hepatitis C, but nothing is yet conclusive. The hep A vaccine consists of two shots over six months, while the hep B vaccine consists of three shots over five to six months. To gain full immunity against hep A or B, you must get all the shots in each series.

*So far, hep A and B are the only sexually transmitted infections that can be prevented with a vaccination. I strongly recommend that all sexually active people who haven't been infected—that probably means you!—be vaccinated against both hepatitis A and hepatitis B.*

**Herpes**

The Centers for Disease Control estimate that as many as 30 million Americans are infected with *herpes,* with half a million new cases occurring each year.[11] Herpes comes in two varieties: herpes simplex virus I and herpes simplex virus II. HSV-I is most often associated with cold sores or fever blisters about the mouth and lips, while HSV-II is associated with sores around the genital area. There's some crossover, however, and each virus will survive quite comfortably in both regions.

## TRANSMISSION

Herpes is generally spread by sexual contact: via intercourse, rubbing genitals together, rubbing the penis on the buttocks, oral–genital contact, anal sex, or rimming. In addition, normally protected areas of skin can become infected if there's a cut, rash, or sore. Herpes viruses can be spread by kissing, if one partner has the infection in or near the mouth. It's possible to transmit the virus even when symptom-free.

## SYMPTOMS

Herpes is marked by clusters of small, painful blisters on the genitals. Some people notice a tingling sensation before blisters appear. After a few days, the blisters burst, leaving small ulcers. In men, the blisters usually appear on the penis, but can appear in the urethra or rectum. In women, they usually appear on the labia, but can appear on the cervix and anal area. First outbreaks are often accompanied by fever, headache, and muscle soreness. First episodes are almost always more severe than recurrences. Blisters are highly contagious. You can spread the virus not only to others but also to other parts of yourself: hands, eyes, and so on. If you touch your blisters, wash your hands thoroughly with hot water and antibacterial soap.

## TREATMENT

There's no medical cure for herpes. Once you have herpes, you have it for life. Treatment with *acyclovir* reduces pain and viral reproduction during outbreaks of sores, although it won't delay or prevent recurrences.

Recurrent sufferers often recognize the first signs of an outbreak (localized tingling, burning, or pain in the genital region) and can begin treatment before blisters appear. This can shorten the cycle and may also reduce the chance of transmission. Immunocompromised people or those who are highly susceptible to repeat attacks (6+ per year) may take a lower daily dose of acyclovir on an ongoing basis as a prophylaxis against outbreaks. Some people find that taking *lysine,* an essential amino acid, prevents or lessens the impact of outbreaks.

### Human Immunodeficiency Virus (HIV)

TRANSMISSION

*HIV* can be transmitted sexually via anal, genital, or oral sexual contact. The risk of transmission varies widely, depending on the type of contact and how infectious a partner is. People with HIV are particularly infectious when they're newly infected—even before an antibody tests registers as positive—as well as in the later stages of illness, when they have AIDS. These are the times when the largest concentration of virus is present. Regardless, it's possible to transmit the virus during a single act of unprotected sex regardless of the infected partner's current stage of disease progression. Statistically, ejaculation into a partner during intercourse is riskier than withdrawal before ejaculation, but withdrawal is a poor prevention strategy because the virus may be present in pre-come in sufficient amounts to infect an HIV-negative partner; besides, transmission from the receptive to the insertive partner is also possible.

Any exposure to a mucus membrane or opening in the skin ups the odds as well. Introducing infected body fluids into the eyes or nose, into open cuts on fingers, or into small sores in the skin caused by concurrent STDs (such as herpes and gonorrhea) probably make it easier to catch HIV—for all of these conditions can provide a passage to the bloodstream.

SYMPTOMS

Most people infected with HIV have no symptoms and wouldn't know they were infected unless they were tested for the presence of antibodies. However, 30% to 70% of newly infected people develop a flu-like illness within two to six weeks of infection.[12] Typically, symptoms last one to two weeks and may include a sore throat, lymph node swelling, muscle aches, night sweats, and a diffuse, flat, red rash over the body. These symptoms resolve on their own.

Shortly after infection, the body begins to hold the virus in check. On average, antibody-positive people remain symptom-free for ten years.[13] So there are a lot of people—*your* potential sex partners, possibly even current ones—who have no idea that they're HIV-positive. During this phase, lymph nodes throughout the body may be swollen and tender. This may be the only symptom of an active infection. Howver, lymph nodes may be swollen for many reasons, and you can't tell from a sexual partner's lymph nodes whether they're infected. A positive result on an HIV antibody test is the *only* way to be sure.

TREATMENT

HIV treatment is one of the most rapidly evolving areas of medical science, but don't fall into the trap of viewing medication as a substitute for safer sex. Taking HIV medication is no guarantee of thwarting HIV's progress. And once you swallow that first set of pills, you're most likely committing to treatment for the rest of your life–a dreary and expensive regimen of rigidly scheduled pill-popping with severe consequences for noncompliance. Skipped dosages may help resistant strains multiply, which could undermine all your efforts at compliance. And in many patients, even when compliance is perfect, HIV eventually develops resistance to their current medications, requiring the patient and doctor to choose from a shrinking pool of alternatives. To complicate matters even further, most of these medications have potential side effects ranging from annoying to severe. Also, the possible ramifications of taking these drugs year after year, such as long-term liver damage, still aren't fully known.

The greatest threat from HIV is its progressive destruction of your natural immunity, which allows cancers and normally harmless opportunistic infections to take hold. If you're HIV-positive, many doctors recommend helping your immune system to remain strong by vaccinating against the following common diseases: hepatitis A and B; diphtheria and tetanus; mumps, measles, and rubella; pneumococcus; and the annual flu vaccine. If you're HIV-positive and sexually active, particularly with multiple partners, it's a good idea to be screened regularly for common STDs as well.

If you're HIV-positive and considering antiviral therapy or alternative treatments, get proactive and do the research. Know what your options are. Acquiring knowledge of current treatment regimens is one way to avoid feelings of helplessness and defeat. By doing their utmost to stay healthy and take control over their destiny, many men have added years to their lives and improved their quality of life and peace of mind immeasurably.

## Parasites and Other Intestinal Infections

Intestinal infections may be caused by bacteria such as *shigella,* by protozoa such as *giardia* (commonly referred to as "parasites" ) or *amoebas* (a/k/a *amebiasis* or *amoebic dysentery*), or by worms such as *thread-worms* or *pinworms*. More than one infection can occur at once. The infectious forms of these germs (bacteria, cysts, or eggs) are found in feces but can survive outside the body for days, so both direct and indirect transmission are possible. In some cases, such as shigella, it takes very little stool to transmit infection. As with hepatitis and bacterial STDs such as syphilis and gonorrhea, intestinal infections are a common consequence of rimming, although some are acquired in foreign travel. Giardia and amoebas are the most common parasites transmitted via rimming, whereas salmonella, shigella, and campylobacter are the most common intestinal bacterial pathogens.

TRANSMISSION
Amoebas reside in your colon, and either they or their reproductive cysts wash out in the stool. The ingested organism grows in the colon. Giardia, on the other hand, resides in the lining of the small intestine and is transmitted via parasitic cysts in feces. Rimming is the most common method of transmission. Fellatio or cunnilingus can also orally introduce parasites into the body when the genital–anal area is contaminated with fecal particulate. Unprotected anal intercourse is also a risk factor, if a man becomes infected from a receptive partner and then has anal intercourse with others. Sharing unsterilized rectal douching equipment is also a possible transmission route.

SYMPTOMS

Most carriers of intestinal infections aren't symptomatic. When symptoms occur, they may be mild or severe, most often including diarrhea, which may contain blood or pus. Additional symptoms include crampy abdominal pain and a low-grade fever. Persistent flatulence (farting) may occur as well.

*Enteritis* is an infection and inflammation of the small intestine, usually caused by giardia or hepatitis A. (In HIV infection, enteritis may also be caused by *cytomegaloviris, MAC, cryptosporidium, isospora,* and salmonella infections.) Symptoms include diarrhea and cramping or abdominal pain, often in the lower left abdomen. Bloating and nausea are often present, too. Diarrhea may be bloody, and there may be a rectal mucus discharge. Fever, chills, general malaise, and even weight loss can also result.

TREATMENT

Amebiasis is diagnosed when a blood test is positive for parasite antibodies or a stool sample reveals the parasite. Giardia is diagnosed via a series of three stool samples, preferably taken on consecutive days. However, even multiple stool samples can be unreliable for giardia, since it lives in the mucus lining, not the stool. If you don't mention your sexual practices to your doctor, he or she may not think of parasitic infection and instead may send you elsewhere for unnecessary tests.

Amoebas and giardia are treated with antibiotics, usually *Flagyl* (metroconizadole). However, Flagyl is a fairly toxic, wide-spectrum antibiotic that kills the good bugs along with the bad ones, so eating yogurt, taking acidophilus capsules, or drinking acidophilus milk to restore intestinal balance is a good idea. Many report mild to extreme discomfort during the treatment period for Flagyl; this seems to be more common in HIV-positive people. Ask about an herbal alternative to Flagyl. An antibiotic (usually Cipro) can treat the bacterial infections salmonella, shigella, and campylobacter, although the bacterial infections usually heal spontaneously with time. Since antibiotic treatment often creates resistant strains, usually it's reserved for those likely to transmit the infection to others, such as through anal sex or food preparation. Unfortunately, relief of symptoms comes earlier than successful treatment, so patients can continue to shed live bacteria and pass infection to others, even though they feel fine.

Three negative stool tests are necessary to confirm successful treatment of any form of intestinal infection. Until then, carriers should assume that they're still capable of infecting others.

## Syphilis

The chronic venereal disease *syphilis* is caused by a bacterium that can infect many different organ systems and lead to a wide range of symptoms. Although antibiotics are effective in treating syphilis, it continues to be a major health problem.

TRANSMISSION
Sexually, syphilis is passed through direct contact between mucus membranes. It can also be transmitted via close skin-to-skin contact, but this is rare. Infection most often occurs during unprotected genital or anal intercourse, although the mouth can also be a site.

SYMPTOMS

Syphilis is sometimes called "the great mimic" since its symptoms often resemble those of other illnesses. A primary-stage *chancre,* or ulcer, on the penis can resemble herpes, and second-stage syphilis has flu-like symptoms. An anal syphilis chancre may be painful and therefore misdiagnosed as a *fissure.* Bloody bowel movements, diarrhea, and mucus discharge are common.

TREATMENT

Penicillin by injection, or a two-week regimen of tetracycline, is the standard treatment for syphilis. Two follow-up blood tests two weeks apart after ending treatment are necessary to ensure successful treatment. Treatment takes longer if the patient has had syphilis for a year or more. In HIV-positive people, higher doses may be required for a prolonged period. Regardless of HIV status, those with syphilis should always be checked for other STDs as well. All sexual partners placed at risk should be notified.

**Venereal Warts**

*Warts* (condyloma acuminatum) are tiny bumps caused by *HPV* (human papilloma virus). The wart is not the actual virus; rather, it's your skin's reaction to it.

TRANSMISSION

Warts may be spread via both sexual and nonsexual means. Unfortunately, warts are very easy to transmit; a wart doesn't need to be present for the virus to spread. Millions of Americans carry the virus and can pass it to sexual partners even if they don't have the warts. Skin-to-skin transmission is sufficient; you don't have to ejaculate or penetrate your partner to spread the virus. Even the hands can transmit HPV from one person's midsection to another's. No one knows why HPV sometimes grows into a wart and sometimes not. Unfortunately, it's next to impossible for a sexually active person to avoid the virus.

SYMPTOMS
Anal warts form in clusters around the anus and sometimes inside the anal canal. They often itch, and friction can cause painful irritation. Venereal warts can also appear on the penis, scrotum, pubic region, buttocks, and inner thighs. Anal warts can also lead to anal fissures (see below). Left untreated, HPV warts may lead to anal cancer.

TREATMENT
Venereal warts can be removed during a visit to the doctor using topical agents, immunotherapy, or surgery. If you have external anal warts, it's important to have an *anoscopy* to check for internal warts as well. (Don't worry; it's a painless procedure.) If your doctor can't or won't perform the anoscopy, find one who will. Do *not* use over-the-counter remedies designed for hand warts; they won't work.

## Anal Sex and Pregnancy

If you have unprotected anal sex with a woman as the receptive partner, you should know that it's not possible to get pregnant that way, because semen can't cross from the anal tract to the vaginal tract *internally*. However, semen leaking from the anus *after* intercourse may drip across the perineum and cause what's colorfully known as a "splash conception."

## Your Anal Health and Well-Being

### Some Parting Thoughts

It's essential to your physical and mental well-being that you find a health care provider with whom you feel comfortable discussing your sexual life. Because of the stigma and denial attached to anal sex, many of us are too embarrassed to discuss it even with our doctors. Yet doing so can make all the difference between suffering in silence from one of the above-described maladies and living a healthy life. In some cases, it's truly a matter of life or death.

Our society separates sex from other aspects of human existence. Most of us have some difficulty in comfortably discussing our sexuality. We compartmentalize it, considering it an unfit topic of conversation in "polite society," and present ourselves to the world with this vital aspect of ourselves glaringly absent.

The only reasonable explanation for this is that we're a sexually fixated culture. Bring up the topic of sex in a typical social setting, and feel how quickly the tension in the room increases. The sexual liberation movement of the 1970s valued sex as a natural and vital part of the range of human experience and expression, yet undue obsession with sex was seen as unhealthy and undesirable.

However, while many proponents of sexual liberation acknowledged this, its implementation has been long in coming, and eludes us still. Sexual topics continue to be a source of embarrassment and discomfort, cloaked in evasions and distortions. With each generation, it seems to get a bit easier, yet many of us still raise our children with few clues as to how sex works and, particularly, what their sexual options are. Many of us still regard sex as a source of awkward giggling and slanderous character defamation, and any mention of a sexually transmitted condition is likely to brand the associated party as a social outcast.

Owing to various societal and interpersonal factors, some of us "go blank" while having sex. This is a fear-based tactic for avoiding responsibility for one's sex life. Many factors can contribute to this behavior, or even increase its likelihood—among them drug consumption, fatigue, the desire to please one's partner, and societal taboos that encourage denial of sexual activity.

It's perhaps even more important in anal intercourse than in other forms of sexual expression to insist on clear communication and complete consciousness. A traumatic experience with anal sex can be difficult to overcome and may impede future enjoyment of sex.

Many of us engage in manipulative and controlling behavior around our sexuality. The more casual sex partners one has, the more likely it is that he or she will encounter such a person. If you feel that you're likely to become a victim of pressure to engage in sexual activities, there are behavior modification courses you can take to curb such pressure. Assertiveness training is one such method; classes are available through many colleges (often the psychology department) and corporate curricula. Copedendence support groups also offer support and hard-won wisdom in the sexual arena.

I have made this statement in so many words elsewhere in this book, but it bears repeating at the end of this chapter on anal health: *You always have the right to say no to anal sex with anyone you feel uncomfortable with*. Whether you're concerned about a prospective partner's lack of integrity, sobriety, awareness about safer sex strategies, or the possibility of their being infected with a sexually transmitted condition, OR ANY-THING ELSE—your sexuality is just that: yours. No one should ever consent to a sexual act because they're feeling pressured to perform, or afraid of losing a partner. Clear, assertive communication is the key to keeping sex hot and safe.

With that in mind, I wish you joy on your erotic journey. Relaxation, communication, and trust—along with lots of lube!—will take you far. Yet there's always more to learn. Be patient, practice with yourself and those you trust, and, by all means, if you discover a new tip or technique, let me know about it! There is always more to learn.

I hope this book brings you closer to the sexual bliss you desire.

## NOTES

1. *Health Care Without Shame*, by Dr. Charles Moser (Greenery Press, 1999).

2. www.bannon.com/kap

3. *Sexually Transmitted Diseases: A Physician Tells You What You Need to Know*, by Lisa Marr, M.D. (Johns Hopkins University Press, 1998), p. 45.

4. Marr, op. cit., p. 129.

5. Marr, op. cit., p. 129.

6. Marr, op. cit., p. 144.

7. "Gonorrhea," www.gayhealth.com/iowa-robot/common/condition.html?record=16

8. Marr, op. cit., p. 121.

9. Marr, op. cit., p. 185.

10. Marr, op. cit., p. 193.

11. www.cdcnpin.org/std/common.htm#herpes

12. Marr, op. cit., p. 232.

13. Marr, op. cit., p. 232.

# 14

# Resources

## BOOKS

*Anal Pleasure and Health,* by Jack Morin (Down There Press, 1998)
- Lays out a comprehensive plan for getting comfortable with anal pleasure.

*The Complete Guide to Safer Sex,* by the Institute for Advanced Study of Human Sexuality, by Ted McIlvenna, M.Div., Ph.D., ed. (Barricade Books, 1999)
- Clearly written, with extensive information and ideas on how to create a safer sex lifestyle.

*The Encyclopedia of Unusual Sex Practices,* by Brenda Love (Barricade Books, 1994)
• Information on lots of things that may give you a few ideas of your own.

*The Ethical Slut,* by Dossie Easton and Catherine Liszt (Greenery Press, 1998)
• How to maintain a nonmonogamous lifestyle.

*The Lesbian S/M Safety Manual,* Pat Califia, ed. (Alyson Publications, 1988, currently out of print)
• Not for lesbians only!

*Sensuous Magic, 2nd edition,* by Patrick Califia (Cleis Press, 2002)
• One of the excellent books on erotic power play targeting a general audience. Back in print and updated after a long hiatus.

*The Strap-On Book,* by A. H. Dion (Greenery Press, 1999)
• A breezy, informal introduction to strap-on play, along with a variety of short fiction pieces illustrating how couples of different orientations and genders can make strap-ons part of their sexual repertoire.

*Trust: The Hand Book,* by Bert Herrman (Alamo Square Press, 1991)
• Dedicated to the sensual art of putting the hand into the butt. The spiritual overtones will repel some but appeal to others.

*The Ultimate Guide to Anal Sex for Women,* by Tristan Taormino (Cleis Press, 1997)
- Hey, just because it's for women doesn't mean it's not also for men! Particularly recommended for men who want to know more about anal sex with women.

*The Ultimate Guide to Strap-On Sex: A Complete Resource for Women and Men,* by Karlyn Lotney (Cleis Press, 2000)
- A comprehensive guide to beginning and advanced topics, in the Ultimate Guide format you're already used to here.

*Urban Aboriginals,* by Geoff Mains (Gay Sunshine Press, 1991, currently out of print)
- Gay male psychological overview of S/M, with lots of anal sex dynamics. A fascinating exploration of erotic power play for all, regardless of gender or orientation.

*The Erotic Mind,* by Jack Morin (HarperPerennial Library, 1996)
- An insightful excursion into sexual psychology by the author of *Anal Pleasure and Health*.

*Good Vibrations: The New Complete Guide to Vibrators, 4th edition,* by Joani Blank and Ann Whidden (Down There Press, 2000)
- The original book on vibrators and related sex toys is now in its fourth edition. Short and concise, this book packs a lot of practical advice into less than 100 pages with humor and style. Oriented toward women but contains some useful information for men as well.

*The Ins and Outs of Gay Sex,* by Stephen E. Goldstone, M.D. (Dell Trade Paperback, 1999)

• Dr. Goldstone's book is a valuable reference containing much useful information designed to combat sexual ignorance among gay men. However, its tone is alarmist at times (forget about douching or fisting!) and occasionally condescending toward the reader. Bear in mind that the author is an M.D. and that doctors sometimes have a rather jaundiced view of sexuality, as they often see the sexual disasters, but not the successes, in their practice.

*Juice: Electricity for Pleasure and Pain,* by Uncle Abdul (Greenery Press, 1998, currently out of print)

*Sexually Transmitted Diseases*, by Lisa Marr, M.D. (Johns Hopkins University Press, 1998)

• This clearly written book begins with excellent discussions of genital anatomy, identifying possible STDs via symptoms, what to expect during an STD exam, how to communicate about sex with a physician or partner, and safer sex. The second half describes the twenty most common STDs in detail. A bit conservative and given to generalization (for example, douching is advised against in *all* circumstances; sex workers are blamed repeatedly and categorically for a high number of infections), but generally you won't go wrong by following Marr's advice.

## MAGAZINES

*Black Sheets,* published (at this point, irregularly) by Black Books, P.O. Box 31155-U, San Francisco, CA 94131, phone (415) 431-0171, fax (415) 431-0172, e-mail BlackSheets@blackbooks.com. $20/4 issues within U.S., $36 outside U.S. "Kinky, queer, intelligent, and irreverent" humorous magazine about sex and popular culture, edited by yours truly. Each issue examines a specific sex-related topic. Some past topics include bisexuality, leather/SM, erotic "drag," sex work, and public sex. At this printing, all seventeen issues are still in print; contact *Black Sheets* for a catalog. Current plans are to expand the magazine into a book series within a year.

*Blue Food,* 1529 W. Lynwood St., Phoenix, AZ 85007, phone (602) 253-2092, www.bluefood.com. At press time, this fun and thought-provoking sex magazine had gone "online only," although all four print issues were still available. Contact for further information.

# VIDEOS

*Bend Over Boyfriend* and *Bend Over Boyfriend 2*
• The first video features sex educators (and real-life partners) doctors Carol Queen and Robert Lawrence. Some of the highlights include demonstrations of Kegel exercises and how to rim safely. The second video is a more straight-ahead anal sex tape. Both are aimed at male/female couples who want to explore male-receptive anal sex, but are appropriate and educational for all orientations.

*Nina Hartley's Guide to Anal Sex*
• This video covers basic anatomy and physiology, as well as "demonstrations" of analingus and other techniques. A good first tape on anal sex.

*Tristan Taormino's Ultimate Guide to Anal Sex for Women, 1 and 2*
• The online catalog at www.blowfish.com describes the first tape as "somewhere between an anal sex instructional video and a butt-soaked raunch-fest." That's about as well as I can do. Butts galore! There's actually some educational value to this tape as well—so get enlightened *and* aroused!

*Rosebud Massage*
• This video is volume 9 in Joseph Kramer's "Gay Wisdom" video series. The master bodyworker shows us five categories of strokes on the anal sphincters (which he calls "the rosebud"): vibrations, stretches, glides, circles, and rotations. He demonstrates on Roger, his lover, more than thirty ways to touch the

rosebud in five different positions with impeccable hygiene. Total nudity.

### Exploring the Land Down Under

• This video is volume 10 of the above series: a talk and demonstration on internal anal massage by Erik Mainard. Mainard shows us a thirty-minute anal massage on his lover, Roger, where the goal is relaxation. Before the massage, Mainard speaks with us about anatomy, self-anal massage, good hygiene, and the use of anal toys.

### Self Anal Massage

• This video discusses breathing, relaxation, self-pleasure with toys, and how to touch the anus. (You'll never think of doorbells the same way again!) There's a certain smugness to this project that's a turn-off, as well as a New Age sensibility that will be grating to some. Internal cleansing is given superficial mention but never explained. Overall, the other tapes seem to cover more concrete, useful information.

# Sources for Anal Fetish Videos

### Video Companies—Men Doing Men

Falcon Studios
P.O. Box 420750, San Francisco, CA 94101,
phone (415) 431-7722 or (800) 227-3717,
www.falconstudios.com/falcon/shoppers.htm.

Hot Desert Knights
100 S. Sunrise Way, #142, Palm Springs, CA 92262,
phone (760) 416-1070 or (800) 300-2002,
fax (760) 416-9304, e-mail bill@hotdesertknights.com;
www.hotdesertknights.com.
• Gay videos and a small sex store. Fisting, bareback-
ing, and water sports videos that are raw and real.
Reasonably priced and very hot. A great place to buy
tapes from a variety of sources as well as HDK's own
great titles. They offer a lot of content for online
viewing, but you must become a member (nominal
$9.95 one-time fee). (reviewed by RedRight)

Hot House Entertainment, Inc.
P.O. Box 410990 #523, San Francisco, CA 94141,
phone (415) 864-8910 or (800) 884-4687,
fax (415) 585-3739, www.hothouse.com.

Kink Video

P.O. Box 420570, San Francisco, CA 94142,

phone (415) 436-9840, fax (415) 436-9840+*51,

www.kinkvideo.com.

- A wide range of fetish videos, including some butt play tapes. The proprietors are fetishists themselves, and they hire amateurs who really love their particular fetish, so the action in Kink Videos is authentic.

Pig Play Products

7985 Santa Monica Blvd., #252,

West Hollywood, CA 90046, phone (213) 656-5170,

fax (213) 715-3600, e-mail pigplayproducts@aol.com;

www.pigplay.com.

- It's pretty clear from their website that they only want to deal directly with retailers. You can try sending an e-mail if you can't find a fetish store near you who carries their videos.

**Mail Order Sources**

Fox Video Mail

P.O. Box 56826, 1040 AV, Amsterdam,

The Netherlands, www.foxvideomail.com.

- Many reasonably priced tape collections worth the money: men fisting men, men fisting women, women fisting men, as well as other fetishes. Save 15% by ordering via registered mail (U.S. cash only, no checks or money orders). Otherwise, order online via PayPal. Free shipping on orders over $100.

VHS Club

P.O. Box 14, Potosi, WI 53820, phone (608) 763-4017.

- Enema/douche lovers: real videos, unusual bags, rubber nurses, doctors, urinary catheterization, showers, medical exams, high volume and essential enemas. Male–male and male–female videos, dominance/submission, piss, and scat videos, and a few specialty items (bags and nozzles) for sale as well. More than 100 items. $4 catalog postpaid. Over a decade of dependable service.

## INTERNET RESOURCES

Anal Health Resources

*Alternative Medicine for Prostate Health*

www.highisland.com/links/index.html

- Links to books on self-help for prostate cancer and informative sites on prostate massage.

*The Daily Apple*

www.thedailyapple.com

- An excellent, informative site. Search on "Prostate Cancer." Fortunately, according to http://my.webmd.com/content/dmk/dmk_summary_account_1452 (see the many links to related articles), prostate cancer is the slowest-growing common cancer, and most men who contract prostate cancer die of other, presumably unrelated, causes.

*Kink Aware Professionals*

www.bannon.com/kap

- Lists physicians, psychotherapists, and other professional service providers who are kink-aware.

*Physical and Mental Health Issues*
www.qrd.org/health
• This page is a collection of articles regarding safer sex for men who have sex with men. The site in general is a huge compendium about everything queer, including history, family, youth, media, politics, sexuality, and more. Unfortunately, it appears that the site hasn't been updated since 1999. Most of the links to external sites are outdated, expired, or forwarded.

*Prostate Cancer From a Patient's Perspective*
www.cooleyville.com/cancer

Patients Helping Other Patients
• Encyclopedic, noncommercial website on prostate cancer, updated daily.

*Prostate Health*
www.menstuff.org/issues/byissue/healthprostate.html
• Useful, informative prostate awareness site (they'll even e-mail you an annual check-up reminder!) with links to recent books on prostate cancer.

*Prostatitis—Pointers to other sites*
www.prostatitis.org/pointers.html

Pointers to Other Sites
• More links.

*Sexual Health Info Center Home*
www.sexhealth.org
- One of the most comprehensive sources of sexual health information on the Internet. A wealth of information and tips on improving your sex life, sex and aging, STDs, and much more. Lots of good basic material on anal sex if you surf a bit through the site— a good place to send Net-surfers who are anal-curious but aren't likely to read this book. A link on the Sex Education Web Circle.

## Anal Sex Resources

*Advanced Anal Sex Techniques*
www.sexuality.org/l/incoming/aanal.html
- This article, by KAZ, provides a very good introduction to anal pleasure. Originally published at www.advancedtechniques.org/anal.html, which links to other interesting articles on cunnilingus, fellatio, and more.

*Anal Sex: A Delicate Decision,* by Cadillac Carter
www.ivillage.co.uk/relationships/sex/sexdil/articles/
0,9546,171_175084,00.html
- "It happens in nearly every lover's lifetime. You'll be asked to do it or you'll want to do it. Whatever your decision, do it safely...."

*Anal Sex: "How To" Guides,* by Sandor Gardos, Ph.D.
http://sexuality.about.com/library/weekly/aa110298.htm
- Suggested guides on anal sex, in print and on the Net.

*Ten Rules of Anal Sex*
www.sexuality.org/l/incoming/analrule.html
- This is a must-read article by Jack Morin, Ph.D., author of *Anal Pleasure and Health*. Not really "rules" for anal sex; rather, this is a list of the ten things most men and women still don't know about anal sex. An excellent primer for novices.

## Curiosities and Miscellanea

*Anal Eroticism: Two Unusual Rectal Foreign Bodies and Their Removal*
www.well.com/user/cynsa/jar.html
- If you ever wanted to know why you shouldn't put strange things up your butt, read this. Weird.

*I Took the Call*
www.well.com/user/cynsa/carrot.html

*Rectal Foreign Bodies*
www.sexuality.org/l/sex/buttobj.html

*Rectal Impaction Following Enema with Concrete Mix*
www.well.com/user/cynsa/cement.html

*Removal of 100-Watt Electric Bulb from Rectum*
www.well.com/user/cynsa/bulb.html

## Fisting/Handballing Resources

*Handball — Gay/Bi Men's Handball (Fisting) Discussion*
www.queernet.org/lists/handball.html
• This is an e-mail list intended for men into handballing. You must subscribe to this one to get their
information; this page is the subscription form.

*Handballing FAQ*
www.sexuality.org/l/sex/hballinf.html
• This is a really short article covering the basics that can
be read as a companion article to the one just above.

*Handballing Guide*
www.sexuality.org/l/sex/handball.html
• This article came from a pamphlet put out by *Trust
Handballing Newsletter*. Avoiding risk, cleaning-out
techniques, comments about urinary tract infection
risks for female fisting bottoms, and more. Some of
my stats on methamphetamine use among handballers came from this site.

*The NEW RedRight Web*
www.winternet.com/~redright/redright.html
• RedRight does a good job of keeping his site current
and, in fact, helped me edit parts of this book. A
FAQ (list of frequently asked questions), links to current fisting sites, photos, fiction, and more. For a
general site directory, go to:
www.winternet.com/~redright/newredright.html.

## General Sexuality Resources

*AltSex.org*

www.altsex.org

- A web site "dedicated to the exploration of the miracle of human sexuality, in all its wonder and diversity." Mostly a directory of links to other specialized sexuality sites, including BD/SM, homosexuality and bisexuality, polyamory, sexual health, transgender issues, and more.

*Charles Haynes' Radical Sex*

www.radical-sex.com

- A jumping-off point for those interested in "radical sexuality" (leathersex and other forms of nonheterosexual-vanilla-variety play). Lots of links and recommendations for further exploration; some are outdated, but it's still a great resource.

*Sexuality.org*

www.sexuality.org/sex.html

- This is the general directory for this comprehensive site, which contains huge amounts of free information on many varied aspects of sexuality. Highly recommended.

## Music

A lot of people like ambient, electronic, or trance music as a background for play. Personally, I don't like music that has a lot of vocals since the words tend to take me out of the intimate space.

Any specific recommendations I make in this regard may soon be out of date, but here are a few of my favorite ambient artists: Mickey Hart, Paul Schütze, Trance Mission, Ray Lynch, and Kitaro. Ambient music with vocals that may work for you are Enya, Enigma, and Dead Can Dance (RedRight calls the first two "almost canonical ass-play music").

Butt Boy composes music specifically for sex; learn more at www.buttboymusic.com. RedRight recommends Conundrum and Cathedral in particular.

Some general suggestions: Try the ambient or New Age section of record stores, or mail-order or online record catalogs. CD stores that cater to disc jockeys have electronic music and all other kinds of interesting stuff. Prowl used record stores if you like to save money. Discs of nature sounds are another possibility. Soundtracks can be a source of music for sex (I'm partial to the Vangelis soundtrack for *Blade Runner,* and I also like the Antonioni soundtrack to certain Fellini movies, as well as Peter Gabriel's *Passion,* which is the soundtrack for *The Last Temptation of Christ*). I have also used classical symphonies and concerti.

*SandMutopian Guardian* (a how-to magazine for fetishists) published three issues (#27, 28, and 29) containing a series of articles by TruDeviant. "Listening in the Dark" includes playlists and descriptions of all kinds of music suitable for play. Issues are $6 each, available for purchase online at www.aswgt.com/UtopiannetworkCOM/1/guardian_bac kissues.htm/. Otherwise, you can contact them at ASWGT, P.O. Box 1146, New York, NY 10156.

Some people enjoy electronic music with a beat, while others dislike any kind of a beat since it can unduly influence their sexual rhythm. And some people find it distracting to have any sort of background music at all. If you don't know your partner's musical preferences, ask before you start playing your Yma Sumac LPs!

## Scat Play Resources

The Internet has become a rallying point for kinky folks who previously had trouble connecting with others who shared their particular fetishes. There are certainly a lot of people on the Internet who are into it or curious! These are the links I found that seemed the most useful to someone who's seeking further information. Note that these sites are X-rated and shouldn't be viewed by anyone under 18 years of age. Sites relating to marginalized sexuality tend to come and go rather quickly, but these two appear to be around for the long haul. I recommend making an online search if you want others.

*RedRight's Scat Site*
www.winternet.com/~redright/scatsite
• An extensive site that includes stories, images, and more, including links to other sites that have useful information on scat play. RedRight (the site host) is compiling a scat FAQ. For a general site directory, go to: www.winternet.com/~redright/redright.html

*Swine-Flu—Health 101 for Pigs*
www.pigmedia.com/health.htm
• Questions regarding scat play, fisting, piss play, enema play, and much, much more are answered here by a board-certified physician with particular knowledge regarding these types of play. For a general site directory, go to www.pigmedia.com/menu.htm.

## SUPPLIES

### Dildos and Butt Plugs

While these are widely available from adult bookstores everywhere, some are better than others, and you usually get what you pay for.

Good Vibrations
938 Howard St., #101, San Francisco, CA 94103, phone (800) BUY VIBE, www.goodvibes.com.
• Good Vibes' product line includes vibrators, dildos ("widest selection of silicone toys available anywhere"), dildo harnesses, hundreds of informational and erotic books, safe sex supplies and information, and a select collection of erotic videos. Free catalog. Very knowledgeable staff that puts you at ease. Clean, well-lighted storefronts in San Francisco and Berkeley.

GreyStar Productions
1750-1 30th St., PMB 608, Boulder, CO 80301,
phone/fax (303) 444-8306. www.bigsextoystore.com
• Wide range of dildos, plugs, vibrators. Many unusual
items including the PostMaster, which uses clamps to
attach your favorite toy to a post for hands-free enjoyment. Also, a mind-boggling and extensive line of Asian
vibrators. Remote control vibrating panties, anyone?

Mercury Mail Order
4077 18th St., San Francisco, CA 94114,
phone (415) 621-1188 or (888) 879-6669,
fax (415) 621-0343, www.mercurymailorder.com.
• MMO features the A to Z of butt toys from small to
huge. A wide variety of dildos, inflatable dildos, plugs,
and many other sex-related goodies. MMO has a catalog ($5) and a San Francisco storefront.

Mr. S Leathers/Fetters
310 7th St., San Francisco, CA 94103,
phone (415) 863-7764 or (800) 746-7677,
fax (415) 863-7798, www.mr-s-leather.com.
• You really need to see the catalog to appreciate the
scope of the Mr. S. product line. They're always coming out with new items—the only way to stay really
abreast is via the online catalog. Among its many
product lines, Mr. S features a wide variety of large
and small butt toys, ranging from teeny-weeny to
enormous. Several lines of butt toys, including the
Creative Mouldings line from the U.K., Domestic
Partners, Square Peg Studios, Falcon, and more.
Storefronts in San Francisco and Los Angeles.

## Custom and Unusual Toys

Cate Cannon
584 Castro St., #815, San Francisco, CA 94114,
phone (510) 235-8475.
• Cate manufactures a line of acrylic butt toys (also available via Mr. S). Their transparency can be rather fun; you can see the pink lining of the rectum by using a flashlight and shining it through the toy.

Divine Interventions
www.divine-interventions.com
• You have to see these people's products to believe them. Functional silicone dildos in the shape of Mary, Jesus on the cross, the Buddha, and more.

Dildos.co.uk
http://dildos.co.uk
• This company is based in the U.K. and deals only with retailers. However, they do provide links to U.S. retailers of their product line, which has some terrific toys in it, all in black! All their toys have men's names, too. This is a fun website with a great attitude toward butt sex. For their list of U.S. retailers, go to www.dildos.co.uk/usa.htm.

Koala Swimwear
P.O. Box 5519, Sherman Oaks, CA 91413,
phone (818) 904-3301 or (800) 238-2941,
fax (818) 780-5170 (recommended for foreign orders),
www.koalaswim.com.
• Exotic and erotic swimwear designs. They offer several thongs and other suits that will hold a butt plug in place: Penetrator, Stimulator, Love Affair, Stimulator Thong, Plug Chaps, Envy, and Tasty are all listed at their website as of this writing.

Mr. S (see above)

- Mr. S. manufactures the "World's Most Comfortable Butt Plug," a metal butt plug in several versions. The most noteworthy aspect of this particular toy is that it tapers to a very thin, rubbery tube connecting the plug to the flange. The user can wear these for hours with no sphincter comfort and still have the filled-up feeling of something in his or her butt. They also make a version that incorporates one or two "bolo" plugs and an aluminum cockring, as well as a version for electroplay. Unique toys, beautifully made, and worth the premium price—I call this line the Cadillac of butt plugs.

Sorodz
Sora Counts, Sorodz, P.O. Box 10692,
Oakland, CA 94610,
phone/fax (510) 482-8252, e-mail info@sorodz.com.

- In addition to her line of whips, rods, paddles, and related S/M paraphernalia, long-time toymaker Sora Counts creates "horse tails," "pig tails," and "feather tails." Good craftsmanship as well as visual and sensual pleasure.

Square Peg Studios
www.douglasstudios.com/squarepeg/
• The entrance page says, "Square peg produces erotic
art objects out of silicone...." The artist here is clearly
a butt pig of major proportions, and his uniquely-
shaped "Crisco-safe" dildos bring together that piggish
desire and a keen aesthetic eye, as well as a genuine
concern for functionality. The first line of silicone toys
to cross over to the male community in a major way.
Offers custom butt toy creation as well as a lifetime
"toy hospital" that will repair your Square Peg silicone
toy free of charge!

Sun Don't Shine Designs
Rudy Bishop, P.O. Box 22472,
San Francisco, CA 94122, phone (415) 753-6711.
• "Custom dildonic engineering," as well as a small
catalog of unusual toys, including some giants in the
shapes of animal phalluses! Send a self-addressed,
stamped envelope for catalog.


**Electrical Toys**

Folsom Electric Co.
584 Castro St., #119, San Francisco, CA 94114,
fax (415) 552-7828, www.folsomelectric.com.
• Get a list of regional dealers throughout the United
States and world from its website. Also offers an
instructional video on electroplay.

Paradise Electro-Stimulations
1509 W. Oakey Blvd., Las Vegas, NV 89102,
phone (702) 474-2991, fax (702) 474-4088,
www.peselectro.com.

**Medical Supplies**

Chase Union, Ltd.
P.O. Box 1014, Novi, MI 48376,
phone (248) 348-8191 or (888) RECTUM1,
fax (248) 348-8394, www.chaseunion.com.
• Medical supplies for the kink community. Rectal spec-
ula, gloves, specialty anal supplies such as anoscopes,
specialty enema supplies such as large-capacity bags
and tanks (including the cylinder device mentioned in
Chapter Four, "Hygiene and Diet"), and lots of really
scary stuff like anal electrodes, "visible ball crusher,"
and "circumcision and castration instruments." Severe
kinkiness combined with attentive service. $2 catalog.

Arthur Hamilton, Inc.
P.O. Box 457, Binghamton, NY 13902,
phone (718) 441-6066 or (888) 783-6937,
fax (718) 441-6066.
• Arthur Hamilton has been around since 1970, keeping enema fetishists well supplied and flushed with
happiness. Among the items in the $2 catalog is an
adjustable stand for an enema bag, medical supplies
such as Chase Union offers, and more. A highly reputable dealer.

High Island Health
P.O. Box 55427, Houston, TX 77255,
phone (713) 721-3611, http://highisland.com.
• Manufacturers of the Pro-State Prostate and Perineal
Acupressure Massager (at this writing, two models,
$40 and $50 plus shipping; add sales tax in Texas).
Their informative website discusses prostate massage
and its benefits.

Klystra
73-1194 Ala Kapua Street, Kailua-Kona, HI 96740,
phone (808) 325-3157 or (800) 708-0477,
fax (808) 325-6326, www.klystra.com.
• Unusual enema supplies for the true fetishist. The
online catalog is quite impressive.

## Safer Sex Supplies (Condoms and More)

Condomania offers a catalog that describes in stunning detail the wide, wonderful world of condoms.
Call (800) 9-CONDOM or visit www.condomania.com.

Good Vibrations sells a condom sampler that includes
five different varieties ($3 at this writing), as well as
details the whole range of condoms. Call (800) 289-
8423 or surf to www.goodvibes.com.

www.managingdesire.org/wheretogetit.html
Where to get it (in bulk): A provider's guide to buying
pregnancy- and disease-prevention supplies
• Condom manufacturers, condom resellers and
repackagers, polyurethane condoms and "female"
condoms, lubricants, oral sex barriers, needle
exchange and outreach supplies, educational materials, outreach worker trainings, and resource and
research information. This site doesn't appear to be
very current (some links are dead), but most of the
toll-free numbers and some of the websites are still in
operation.

J-lube
Nasco, 4825 Stoddard Rd., Modesto, CA 95356,
phone (209) 545-1600 or (800) 558-9595,
fax (209) 545-1669, www.nascofa.com/prod/home.
 • The item number is C08175N at $9.50 for 8 oz. of the
   powder, which makes six to eight gallons of the
   strange stuff, which is used primarily in the kinky community by fisters. It takes a lot less J-lube to fist someone than it does to deliver a calf! In other words, you
   don't want to mix this package all at once. *NOT a sex-
   toy company, so it pays to be discreet.* You can also
   purchase J-lube via Mr. S.


## Slings and Furniture

Custom furniture and equipment for sex is still largely a
cottage industry, and sometimes it takes craftspersons a
while to fill your order. Whether this is due to the exacting nature of the order, the unfortunate tendency for
crafters to be swamped with requests, or general flaki-
ness on the part of a specific individual is for you to
determine. Patience and clear communication on the
part of both parties benefits all.

BDG Sales
P.O. Box 100589, Milwaukee, WI 53210,
phone (414) 871-9270 or (cell) (414) 559-2347,
fax (414) 871-9277, www.BDGsales.com.
 • Dungeon furniture. Slings, bondage tables, and more,
   including a spanking bench with tie-down straps that
   makes a great bench for anal sex and oral sex, too.

Dungeon Enterprises
P.O. Box 35854, #644, Dallas, TX 75235,
phone/fax (214) 522-2796,
www.dungeon-enterprises.com.

• Suppliers of unusual kinky merchandise including nitrile gloves in quantities as small as a single box. Slings (portable and stationary), restraints, rubber sheets, electronic dog collars, electric boxes, shackles, enema supplies, grease guns ((yikes!)), and much more.

JIMsupport Enterprises
757 Williams Rd., Palm Springs, CA 92264,
phone (760) 416-9315, fax (760) 416-9273,
http://jimsupportportasling.homestead.com/portasling.html.

• A respected supplier for stand-alone slings (self-contained with frame) is JIMsupport, maker of the Porta-Sling. According to RedRight, their product is "first rate and they are great to deal with. I have done extensive testing, and this is really the best portable sling you can get."

Also, Mr. S and most major leather shops, as well as some sex toy stores such as Good Vibrations, have various forms of sex furniture available.

## Sex Information Hotlines

American Social Health Association  Hotlines:
CDC National STD & AIDS Hotlines
(800) 342-2473 or (800) 227-8922 – English
(800) 344-7432 – En Español
(800) 243-7889 – TTY (Deaf access)

National Herpes Hotline
(919) 361-8488

San Francisco Sex Information
(877) 472-7374, (415) 989-SFSI (California)
Free, volunteer-run   information and referral switch-
board providing anonymous, accurate, non-judgmental
information about sex.

## About the Author

BILL BRENT is a San Francisco writer, editor, and publisher. He spent two years as a shift supervisor for San Francisco Sex Information. He is the editor of *The Black Book*, the resource guide to alternative sexuality and, with Dr. Carol Queen, co-editor of *Best Bisexual Erotica* (Black Books). His fiction has appeared in *Best American Erotica, Best Gay Erotica, Noirotica, Rough Stuff,* and *Touch Guys* (which he co-edited with Rob Stephenson). You can reach him at BB@blackbooks.com.